QUICK EASY KETOGENIC COOKING

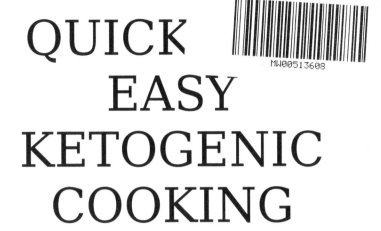
The Fast Track To Epic Health And Wellness Living

DIANA WATSON

BOOK ONE

KETOGENIC DIET FOR BEGINNERS

Simple and Fun 3 Weeks Diet Plan for the Smart

DIANA WATSON

Table of Contents

VIP Subscriber List

Hi Dear Reader, this is Diana! If you like my book and you want to receive the latest tips and tricks on cooking, weight-loss, cookbook recipes and more, do subscribe to my mailing list in the link here! I will then be able to send you the most up-to-date information about my upcoming books and promotions as well! Thank you for supporting my work and happy reading!

Introduction

Congratulations on purchasing *Ketogenic Diet for Beginners: Simple and Fun 3 Weeks Diet Plan for the Smart* and thank you for doing so. The following chapters will discuss what exactly the ketogenic diet is and how it can help you improve your life, whether it be from weight loss or a boost in energy. The benefits of the ketogenic diet are immense, which means you too can start to make a powerful and wise lifestyle change.

There are plenty of books on this subject on the market, thanks again for choosing this one! Every effort was made to ensure it is full of as much useful information as possible, please enjoy!

Chapter 1: How It Works

There are so many different diet plans out there, it can be confusing and overwhelming when you are deciding which one would work best for you. Some of these diets are trends or fads and not something that can be maintained long-term, others might make you feel hungry all the time, which as you know, does not make for a happy life. This is one of the reasons the ketogenic diet stands apart from the rest, it will help you lose weight, while also letting you feel satisfied. You are not starving your body of calories or fat on the ketogenic diet.

What Does Ketogenic Mean?

When you eat a more traditional diet that is higher in carbohydrates your body produces glucose and insulin. Glucose is the body's first choice of energy source because it is the easiest for the body to convert. Insulin's role is to process the glucose that is in your bloodstream by taking it around the body. When this happens, it means that the fats in your body are not needed, since they are not the energy source. The fat still has to go somewhere though, so the body stores it for later use.

When you lower your carbohydrate intake, your body will enter into a state known as ketosis, which is where the word ketogenic comes from. Ketosis is what the body initiates when food consumption is low, it is a natural process that is meant to help the body survive. During ketosis the liver will break down fats and produce ketones which can also be used as fuel for the body, but only if glucose is in short supply. Remember, glucose is the body's first choice, so it will only use something else when glucose is not an option. It is not because it can't or that is not healthy, when using ketones as fuel, the body just has to work a little harder.

The goal of the ketogenic diet is to get your body to switch from using glucose as its fuel supply, to ketones, which you would get from the breakdown of fat. Therefore, your body would be getting all its energy from fat. As your insulin levels lower, your body's fat burning abilities will increase. For most people, this happens very quickly and quite dramatically. One of the benefits of this diet is how easy it becomes to burn through stored fat, which obviously helps if weight loss is your main goal.

The quickest way to enter ketosis is by fasting, however that cannot be maintained without harmful effects. The ketogenic diet can be followed indefinitely, while still allowing the body to enter ketosis. This is not a diet that deals with calorie counting, meaning you cannot eat what ever you want as long as you don't go over your caloric limit. Keeping your carbohydrate intake low, it is suggested no more than 20 or 30g of net carbohydrates is how you will be successful. However, the less you consume, the more dramatic your weight loss will be.

What is a Net Carb?

Net carb = Total dietary carbohydrate – Total fiber

Let's assume you want to eat one cup of broccoli, which contains 6g of total carbohydrates and 2g of fiber. To find the net carbs, you would then take the 6g minus the 2g, leaving you with 4g, which is the net carb amount.

Your ketogenic diet should be made of around 70

percent fats, 25 percent proteins, and only 5 percent should be carbohydrates. This is why it is so important to pay attention to what you are putting into your body and whether or not it will prevent you from entering ketosis.

The ketogenic diet will yield impressive results, but only if you stick to it. When you eat too many carbohydrates, your body will have the insulin it needs to use as fuel, meaning the fat will be stored instead of burned. The secret to a successful ketogenic diet is to plan-out what you will eat, this will not only reduce your stress, but it will also keep you on the right track.

Just like any diet or lifestyle change, it will take time for you to properly adjust to it, but you can do it. One of the best things you can do for yourself is to keep an open mind and allow yourself the time necessary to acclimate. Rushing things before you are fully prepared will not help you, it will only cause you added stress which will probably lead to failure. To prevent this from happening, it is crucial that you find what works for you while still adhering to the diet.

Some people prefer to prep their meals a head of time, especially breakfast and lunch since they often take it with them to work. Other people like to write out their meals like a menu and stick with their ideas. You don't have to do this, but it definitely make things easier on you, especially in the beginning.

When you are on a special diet like this one, it probably won't take you very long to see how much easier it is to cook at home. Being in complete control of your food is crucial to remaining in ketosis and losing weight. That being said, if you do decide to go to a restaurant, make sure to ask any appropriate questions involving your order. Being specific about what foods are cooked in or how they are prepared will help make sure you are sticking to your diet.

Just remember, you are not going to be hungry, your body is learning to depend a different fuel for energy. That takes some time to get accustomed to, so be patient with yourself and find what works best for you. For instance, if you prefer to prep all of your meals for the week on Sunday, do it. However, if you work the night shift and enjoy cooking when you arrive home in the morning, feel free to do it that way, just find what works for you and stick to it.

Chapter 2: All About Food

Starting a new diet can be frustrating and irritating, especially if you think you are sticking to the rules, but are not seeing any positive results. This is why it is so important to know exactly what you are allowed to eat what you are not. If you don't know what foods are acceptable and are not knowledgeable about your diet, you won't be successful, regardless of the effort you are putting forth. So, make it easy on yourself and learn which foods you should eat and which you should avoid.

The best way to think of the ketogenic diet is to think real, whole foods. Anything that is prepackaged or processed is full of net carbohydrates and is off limits. This means staying away from pastas, cereals, breads, and cakes. Fruits and vegetables also contain carbohydrates so it is important that you also keep track of these net carbs as well. You already know that your diet is going to consist of mostly healthy fats, but you might understand what that means exactly. Well, first, not all fats are equal, some are definitely better for you than others and it is crucial that you know the difference.

Fats, Good and Bad

Foods contain different types of fats, but are categorized by what they contain the most of. For instance, butter is considered a saturated fat because it contains 60 percent saturated fat. As you move forward with your diet you will quickly understand the role fats play, without them you would be hungry all the time and would be left feeling unsatisfied.

Saturated Fats – These are known as essential to our health as they help to keep our immune systems healthy. In addition to helping with the immune system, this fat will also help balance hormone levels and maintain a normal bone density. This type of fat has a bad reputation and time and again has been included in the 'bad for you' category, but many different studies have shown that they are important and necessary for a healthy body. Meats, butter, and eggs all have saturated fats in them.

Polyunsaturated Fats – This is the type of fat that is commonly found in vegetable oils, and for a long time they were thought to be beneficial. However, that is not the case as they are often over processed, for instance, "heart healthy" margarines have been linked to heart disease. Yet, polyunsaturated fats that are natural such as those found in fish actually help to lower cholesterol, so it is important to know the difference and not get them confused. This is why real, natural foods are so important because the fats they contain are much better for you than their highly processed counterparts.

Monounsaturated Fats – This is an accepted healthy fat, as it improves insulin resistance and cholesterol levels. This type of fat is found in both sunflower and olive oils, both of which are common and easy to incorporate into your diet.

Trans Fats – You probably already know that trans fats are not good for you, they do not occur in natural fatty foods, only processed fatty foods. That is an important distinction, because this type of fat is created from chemicals that are used to extend a food's shelf-life. For instance, the hydrogenation process is when hydrogen is added to these fats which changes their chemical make-up. Even if a label does not say it contains trans fats, if it says hydrogenated on it, avoid it.

When you are doing your grocery shopping, try to purchase organic products and grass-fed proteins. Avoid canned or frozen fruits and vegetables too, but it is understandable that some people just do not have the financial means to do this, so be cautious and make sure you read all the labels. The next chapters are going to contain some recipes that you can try, but as you progress with your diet, you will see how easy it is to incorporate healthy fats into your meals. This will help you feel satisfied and will help you stay fuller longer.

Fats:
Avocado
Beef Tallow
Chicken Fat
Macadamia Nuts

Ghee

Butter

Non-hydrogenated Lard

Mayonnaise – read the label and make sure it does not have added carbs.

Red palm oil

Peanut butter

Olive oil

Coconut oil

Proteins:

Fish – Try to purchase wild caught if available, this can include salmon, trout, catfish, halibut, cod, flounder, mackerel, tuna, and snapper.

Shellfish – Crab, oysters, mussels, squid, lobster, scallops, and clams.

Whole Eggs – Opt for free-range if you can, local organic farmers often have them cheaper than your local grocery stores. When it comes to preparation you have many different options such as boiled, poached, scrambled, deviled, and fried.

Meat – Grass-fed typically has a higher fatty acid count, so opt for grass-fed when given the opportunity. Goat, lamb, veal, beef, and other wild game are all good choices.

Pork – You can eat nearly any type of pork, just make sure to read the label to make sure there are no added sugars.

Poultry – Pheasant, quail, chicken, and duck are all acceptable, but choose free range and organic if it is possible.

Sausage and Bacon – This can still be an acceptable and even beneficial protein as long as you choose it wisely, make sure there are no extra fillers and that it is not cured in sugar.

Peanut Butter – Choose natural peanut butter, but make sure to read the label carefully, even the most natural peanut butter can contain high amounts of carbohydrates, a better alternative is macadamia nut butter.

Vegetables

The best vegetables to eat on the ketogenic diet are those that are leafy and grow above ground. Again, if you can eat organic, try to do so as there will less pesticides used in the growing process, but if you can't try not to worry too much. Studies have shown that both non-organic and organic vegetables have the same nutritional qualities.

Of course vegetables are good for you, but some are better than others in terms of the ketogenic diet. For instance, some vegetables are high in sugar and lower in important nutrients, these are the types of vegetables that you want to either cut out altogether or consume only in very small portions. The best vegetables for this diet are those that are low in carbohydrates and high in nutrients, such as kale and anything green leafy that resembles it. These types of veggies are also easy to include in meals and they really pack a powerful nutrition punch as well.

Remember, vegetables also contain carbohydrates, so make sure you are keeping track throughout the day so you stay well within the acceptable limit. The following is a list of vegetables and their net carbohydrates by ounce.

Avocado - .6

Broccoli – 1.1

Baby Carrots – 1.5

Cauliflower - .5

Celery - .3

Cucumber – 1

Green Beans – 1.3

Mushrooms - .6

Green Onion – 1.3

White Onion – 2.1

Green Pepper - .8

Romaine Lettuce - .3

Butterhead Lettuce - .3

Shallots – 3.9

Snow Peas – 2.8

Spinach - .4

Acorn Squash – 2.9

Butternut Squash – 2.1

Spaghetti Squash – 1.4

Tomato - .8

As you begin making your own meal plans, simply

add up the net carbohydrates between the different foods so you have an idea of how many you are consuming from that meal. This will get easier over time, you can even try writing it down in the beginning until you get more comfortable keeping track.

Dairy

Dairy products are also acceptable as long as there is no added sugars or other additives. It is best to go choose full fat, raw, and organic.

Sour Cream

Cottage Cheese

Heavy Whipping Cream

Hard and Soft Cheeses (Cream cheese, cheddar, mozzarella, mascarpone, etc)

You probably are guessed what is going to be said next, but it really can't be stressed enough, make sure you read the labels. Many cheeses are low in net carbohydrates as it is, but if you are in doubt either read the label or as the person behind the counter.

Nuts and Seeds

Seeds and nuts are a great way to add healthy fats to your diet and make a wonderful and convenient snack. It is best to eat them when they are roasted, this process removes any anti-nutrients. It is also important to note that there is a difference between a nut and a legume, nuts are allowed, while legumes are generally not permitted. Oddly enough, based on the name, a peanut is a legume and should be avoided. Here is a list of acceptable nuts and seeds:

Macadamias, walnuts, and almonds, all of these should be eaten in moderation, but their carbohydrate count is relatively low.

Pistachios and cashews are both higher in carbohydrates, but do contain healthy fats, so make sure you keep careful track of them.

Tip: Seed and nut flower are good alternatives to white or wheat flour, but try not to make this a staple in your diet because nuts are high in Omega-6 fatty acids, so be careful with over eating them because it can lead to weight gain and slow your progress.

Beverages

When you start your ketogenic diet, you will notice

that it will have a natural diuretic effect, which means hydration is even more important. Also, if you are someone who is prone to bladder pain or urinary tract infections, you will need to be even more diligent when it comes to hydrating. It is suggested that you not only drink the recommended eight glasses of water each day, more in addition. Our bodies are made up of 2/3 water, so make sure you are keeping it happy and hydrated. Drink appropriate liquids like it is going out of style!

Water, drink it. Drink a lot of it.

Coffee, with heavy cream and no sugar, it is fine in moderation.

Tea, also no added sugar and if you like it with milk make sure it is raw and whole fat or use heavy cream.

Sweeteners

Of course it is best to avoid anything that is sweet, but for some of us with a sweet tooth, this would just make us miserable. That being said, if you have a sweet craving that you can't seem to deny, choose an artificial sweetener and try not to do this often. Liquid sweeteners are better since there are no added binders like in the powder forms that have carbohydrates.

Stevia

Sucralose

Monk Fruit

Erythirol

Xylitol

Spices

When it comes to what you eat, you want it to be flavorful and satisfying, most of which will come from the addition of spices. However, many spices contain carbohydrates, so it is important that you keep track of the amounts of you are using and add those amounts to your carbohydrate total for your meal. You can use nearly any dry spices you prefer, just make sure you look up the carbohydrate content, no one wants your food to be boring and bland. Some spices have more carbs than others, such as cinnamon, garlic powder, allspice, bay leaves, ginger, and cardamom, so if those are staples in your cooking, make sure you are keeping accurate track.

Watch Out For

Fruit – Limit your fruit content because fruit is high in natural sugars and therefore carbohydrates. Many people use berries in desserts or as snacks, but only in small portions and not very often. If you choose to do this, be cautious of raspberries, cranberries, and blueberries.

Tomato – Food companies are very good at making their products look healthier than they really are. Tomatoes do have natural sugars in them, but when you buy tomato based products additional sugar is often added. That doesn't mean you can't use canned tomato sauces or diced tomatoes, just make sure you read the labels.

Peppers – Most of us do not think of peppers as being full of sugars, green has the last amount of sugars compared to red or yellow.

Diet Sodas – You can still drink diet soda, just pay close attention to how much you are drinking and try to limit yourself if you are soda dependent. Some people have reported that they were knocked out of ketosis from consuming too much artificial sweetener, so just keep that in mind when you are considering a diet soda.

Salt – Since the ketogenic diet acts as a natural diuretic, you will see that your body does not retain salt the same way it did before. This means that salt and other electrolytes are flushed from the body very quickly, this can lead to many different health issues such as panic attacks and heart palpitations. To prevent this from happening you can include salted bone broth into your diet or you can use what is known as a light salt that is a combination of both salt and potassium. Most people also choose to take a supplement for anything they think are not getting enough of from their diet.

Water – When you think you have consumed enough water, drink a little more. Your body is going through some huge changes and part of that is flushing out liquids faster than before, so to keep yourself healthy it is a good idea to drink water, a lot of water.

In The Beginning

If this your first time embarking on a low carbohydrate diet, there are some things you need to know. Your body is doing to go through what is known as detox symptoms, this is perfectly natural, but uncomfortable. Remember, you are retraining your body, that doesn't happen without consequences. However, don't be discouraged, they only last for a few days and no matter how bad it feels, you can and will get through it.

These withdrawal symptoms are commonly referred to as the "keto flu," which sounds much worse than it is. Just keep telling yourself that the first three days are the hardest and it will get much easier after. Here is a list of the symptoms:

Irritability

Fatigue

Dizziness

Intense Cravings

Basically, your body is acting like an unruly child who wants sugar, because it has become so accustomed to it. For those who are transitioning from a very carbohydrate dense diet the symptoms will be much worse than others, it just depends on the person's body. Just don't give up. There are some things you can do to help cope with the negative side effects by increasing your water intake. When the very intense cravings hit, and they will, give your body something to eat, just not what it wants, try bacon or cheese. You are not denying yourself food, just distracting it from craving carbohydrates, until you adjust, distraction is the key to success.

Benefits

Now that you just read about the negative side effects, you might be feeling even more overwhelmed than before. However, the benefits of the ketogenic diet far outweighs the negative. Here is a list of the benefits:

Less appetite - After your body has had time to adjust to ketosis, your appetite will just naturally be reduced. This will also eventually lead to less calorie intake too.

Weight Loss - Not only will you lose weight on this

diet, but not all fat is the same. When you hold more fat in the abdominal area, this can cause many different health issues, even increasing your risk of heart disease. The ketogenic diet will help you lose weight in the abdominal area, and usually rather quickly, this will help those who are risk for type 2 diabetes as well as heart disease.

Blood Pressure – The ketogenic diet helps to reduce high blood pressure and is often suggested by doctors for this reason.

The Brain – Some parts of the brain can only use glucose which is why our liver will create glucose from protein when we do not eat carbohydrates. However, most of the brain is capable of using ketones as fuel. Allowing the brain to use ketones as fuel has helped many children and adults alike with epilepsy. Currently, scientists are looking into a connection between the ketogenic diet and Alzheimer's disease.

Now, you have an idea of what you are going to be eating and how to count the net carbohydrates in the foods. When you first start out, keep very close track of your portion sizes so you can keep an accurate record of the net carbs. If you are choosing to remain under 20 net carbohydrates a day, then make sure to include not only the ingredients from the meal you are eating, but also from the beverage and even the spices. You will want to do this for each meal so you know for sure you are not exceeding your limit.

This is probably not going to come very easily in the beginning, but rest assured, it will get easier for you. Also, after you stick to the diet for a couple of weeks, you will already start to see results and nothing works to motivate quite like seeing the desired results. Even if it feels like you just can't keep going, or you want to give up, don't, it was hard for nearly everyone in the beginning. You are going through something huge, retraining your brain and learning to control your cravings. Chances are, you are also breaking some bad habits as well, so give yourself the necessary time to fully adjust.

Chapter 3
Ketogenic Breakfasts

This is a collection of ketogenic recipes that you can mix and match to give you a three week jump start on your diet. This will help you by taking the guess work out of what to make and it will also give you a general idea of how to prepare the correct foods for yourself. Once you start your new diet, you might find that you choose to meal prep for the week, and if that is the case, make sure your choices are able to be stored appropriately.

Many people think breakfast is one of the hardest meals to create because you can only eat so many eggs and bacon before you are craving variety. For that purpose, traditional eggs and bacon or sausage are going to be avoided, in favor of other easy and more creative options.

Egg Porridge

1/3 cup heavy cream

2 eggs

Cinnamon to taste

2 tablespoons butter

Berries, optional

Sweetener, optional

This is a ketogenic version of oatmeal or porridge, it is based on how eggs curdle and uses that grainy feel as added texture. You can choose whether or not to add berries or sweetener, depending on how many carbohydrates you are allotting yourself.

1. Combine the cream, eggs, and sweetener if you choose to use it in a small bowl and whisk the mixture together until uniform in color.
2. In a saucepan melt the butter over medium-high heat, but keep an eye on it and do not

allow it to turn brown. Once the butter is melted, turn the heat to low.

3. Add the cream and egg mixture to the butter in the saucepan, make sure you continue mixing, especially along the bottom because that is where it will start to curdle and thicken first. Once you start to see the little grains or curdles remove it from the heat.

4. Add a serving to a bowl and sprinkle the top with cinnamon and the berries if you choose.

5.

6. Cream Cheese Pancakes

7. 2 eggs

8. ½ teaspoon cinnamon

9. 2 ounces of cream cheese (read the label and make sure there are no added sugars)

10. 1 teaspoon sweetener, optional

11. Butter, to grease pan

12. You will also need a blender or a food processor for this recipe.

13.

1. Place all the ingredients into the blender or food processor and mix until smooth. Sit it aside and allow it to rest for two or three minutes, or until the bubbles are settled.
2. Grease the pan and set it on medium high heat, with the butter and pour the batter onto the pan, just like you would with traditional pancakes. Cook for two minutes and then flip, cook for an additional minute or until golden brown. Repeat this until all of the batter has been used.
3. You can eat these with sugar-free syrup, berries, or nothing at all depending on what your carbohydrate limit is.
4.
5. This is a great recipe to make for large groups since it is so easy and quick. They will make a great addition to your diet and will leave you feeling full and satisfied.
6.
7. **Lemon Poppy Seed Muffins**
8. 2 tablespoons poppy seeds
9. Zest of 2 lemons
10. 3 tablespoons lemon juice

11. 3 large eggs

12. ¾ cup almond flour

13. ¼ cup flaxseed meal

14. 1 teaspoon vanilla extract

15. ¼ cup heavy cream

16. 1/3 cup erythritol

17. 1 teaspoon baking powder

18. ¼ salted butter, melted

19. 25 drops of liquid sweetener

20. Muffin pan and liners

21.

1. Set your oven to 250F, and in a bowl combine the flaxseed meal, poppy seeds, almond flour, and erythritol.

2. Slowly pour in the eggs and heavy cream, stir constantly until the mixture is smooth and there are no lumps in the batter.

3. Once the mixture is smooth add the sweetener, vanilla extract, lemon juice, lemon zest, and baking powder. Make sure to stir this well to ensure everything is mixed together properly.

4. Put your liners in the muffin pan, or silicone molds, this batter will make 12 muffins, but if

you need to you can adjust the size a little, just try not to make them too big.

5. Place your batter in the oven and bake for 18 to 20 minutes, if you want a crispier crust on the bottom, leave them in for a bit longer.

6. When they are finished baking, take them out of the oven and let them rest on the counter for around 10 minutes.

7.

8. These are the perfect breakfast for people who want something they can easily take with them. If you know you are in for a busy week, these make for a great breakfast to make before your work week starts.

9.

10.

11. 'McGriddle' Casserole

12. 10 eggs

13. 1 cup almond flour

14. ¼ cup flaxseed meal

15. 1 pound breakfast sausage

16. ½ teaspoon onion powder

17. ½ teaspoon garlic powder

18. ¼ teaspoon sage

19. 4 tablespoons sage

20. 4 ounce cheddar cheese

21. 6 tablespoons sugar free syrup

22. Salt and pepper to taste

23. Casserole pan

24. Parchment paper

25.

1. Preheat the oven to 350F and put a pan on medium heat, this is for the breakfast sausage. You are going to break it up as you brown it.

2. In a large mixing bowl combine all of the dry ingredients, mix them together and then add the wet ingredients, but only put in 4 tablespoons of the syrup. Mix everything together until is uniform and smooth.

3. After your mixture is mixed well, add the cheese and stir some more.

4. Throughout this process, you should also be checking on your sausage to make sure it is not getting too brown, you just want it to be a little crispy. When it is cooked to your liking, pour it, with the fat, into the mixture and stir everything together.

5. Place the parchment paper into your casserole pan and pour the mixture into the dish. Drizzle the remaining syrup over the top of the mixture.

6. Bake for about 45 to 55 minutes, if your pan is larger and your casserole thinner, you will need to adjust the cooking time to a bit less. You want the inside to be cooked through completely though, you'll know it is when it is golden brown and looks firm.

7. When it is done cooking, remove it from the oven and gently pull out the parchment paper, slice the casserole into pieces and serve with either sugar-free ketchup, or even a little more syrup.

8.

9.

10.

11. This is a great recipe that you can eat all week. Feel free to alter the recipe to suit your needs, for instance, if you think it is too much syrup, you can adjust the amount.

12.

13. Breakfast Tacos

14. 6 eggs

15. 3 strips of bacon

16. ½ avocado

17. 1 cup shredded mozzarella, make sure it is whole milk

18. 1 ounce shredded cheddar cheese

19. 2 tablespoons butter

20. Salt and pepper to taste

21.

1. First, you are going to cook the bacon, the easiest way is to preheat your oven to 375F and bake it for 15 to 20 minutes, but if you choose to cook it in a pan, that's fine too.

2. While the bacon is cooking, put 1/3 of a cup of mozzarella in a clean pan on medium heat. You want it to be uniform in thickness and in a circle, this is what will be your taco shell. Be patient, this takes some practice to get right, but you'll get the hang of it.

3. After about two or three minutes the edges will be brown, this is when you are going to carefully slide a spatula underneath it. If you used whole milk mozzarella this should be

easy since the oils in it prevent it from sticking naturally.

4. Rest a wooden spoon over a large bowl, using either tongs or your spatula, gently drape the mozzarella over the spoon so as it hardens it will be in the shape of a crunchy taco shell. Do this to the rest of the mozzarella, which will leave you with three completed shells when finished.

5. Your next step is to cook your eggs in the butter, you can do a soft or a hard scramble, it's your preference.

6. When your eggs are finished, spoon them into each of your taco shells and add the sliced avocado on top. Then top with our bacon, you can simply place the entire slice on each, or dice it up.

7. The final step is to sprinkle the cheddar cheese on each taco and enjoy.

8.

9. This is a breakfast that helps people transition when they are craving that crunch that carbohydrates provides. So, if you find yourself craving chips or breads, this might

help satisfy you. Keep in mind though, that even though these do not take too long to make, they are not like the casserole where you can make extra for the week. You are pretty much just making a serving at a time.

10.

11. Brownie Muffins

12. ¼ cup cocoa powder

13. 1 cup flaxseed meal

14. ½ tablespoon baking powder

15. 1 egg

16. 1 tablespoon cinnamon

17. 2 tablespoons coconut oil

18. ½ teaspoon salt

19. ½ can pumpkin puree

20. ¼ tsp sugar-free caramel syrup

21. 1 teaspoon apple cider vinegar

22. ¼ cup slivered almonds

23. 1 teaspoon vanilla extract

24.

1. Preheat your oven to 350F and put all the dry ingredients into a large mixing bowl.

2. In a separate mixing bowl combine all the wet ingredients and stir until uniform and smooth.

3. Gently pour the wet ingredients into the dry bowl and mix together until everything is smooth and it is smooth.
4. Put your muffin liners into your pan and spoon about ¼ cup of batter into each one, and sprinkle the almonds over the top, press them down slightly so they don't fall off. This recipe will make 6 muffins, if you need 12, simply double all of the ingredients.
5. Place them in the oven and check on them after about 15 minutes, you will know they're done when they rise. You can eat them either cold or warm, they make the perfect addition to your morning coffee.

6.
7. This is the perfect breakfast for anyone who has a sweet tooth. So, for those who are starting a low carbohydrate diet for the first time, these can help with those intense sweet carb cravings. You should not feel hungry and unsatisfied on your diet and this is a great way to make sure that doesn't happen.
8.

9. These breakfasts can be mixed and matched throughout the weeks, or you can make the casserole and eat it for the whole week. You can even freeze individual servings and microwave it when needed. You want your diet to work around your life, not change your life to work around your diet. Too many huge changes at one time can lead to failure. So, find what meals work for you and stick to it, for instance, if you are more likely to hit the snooze button on your alarm and find yourself rushing, setting aside time to cook an elaborate breakfast, might not be feasible. If that is the case, the casserole or the muffins would be best for you.

10.

11.

12.

13.

14.

15.

16.

17.

18.

19.

20.

21.

22.

23.

24.

25.

26. Chapter 4

27. Ketogenic Lunches

28.

29. When it comes to ketogenic friendly foods, it is usually best if you prepare them at home so you know exactly what you're eating. If you have a tendency to go out to lunch when you are at work, bringing it might seem strange in the beginning. However, it is easier than trying to find ketogenic friendly foods on a menu that does not usually have them specifically listed. Going out to eat can be frustrating because you will need to ask the server so many different questions about ingredients. Until you are more comfortable and confident with your diet, it is a good idea to bring your lunch with you, just to ensure that you remain in ketosis.

30.

31. Just like with the breakfasts, you can make your lunches daily if you choose, or you can prep things a head of time. Some people prefer to only make lunches that can frozen in individual servings so all they have to do is thrown the Tupperware into their lunchbox and be on their way. Others prefer to prepare their lunch night before or their morning of work, depending on time and what they are in the mood for. The following recipes are all easy and quick, and fit well with the mix and match three week plan.

32.

33. Mixed Green Salad

34. 3 tablespoons roasted pine nuts

35. 2 tablespoons shaved parmesan

36. 2 ounces of mixed greens

37. 2 slices of bacon

38. Salt and pepper to taste

39. Ketogenic friendly dressing of your choice, read the label carefully

40.

1. Cook the bacon until it is crispy, you can do this the oven or in a pan, it is up to you. Some people prefer to burn the edges just a bit to add bitter notes to the salad, this complements vinaigrette dressings especially well.
2. Put your portioned greens into a container that has a lid with some extra room, this is for shaking purposes, so keep that in mind when choosing.
3. Crumble the bacon into the greens and toss in the rest of the ingredients including the dressing. Put the lid on the top and shake the container until the dressing coats the greens evenly.

4.
5. If you are taking this with you to work, wait until you get to work to combine the ingredients. You can keep them separate in reusable bags or in small containers. This helps to keep the salad from getting soggy.
6.
7. Pigs in a Keto Blanket
8.

9. 37 small sausages, read the label carefully

10. 1 egg

11. 1.5 ounces of cream cheese

12. 8 ounces of cheddar cheese

13. ¾ almond flour

14. 1 tablespoon psyllium husk powder, or coconut flour

15. Salt and pepper to taste

16.

1. Combine all the dry ingredients in a large bowl.

2. Melt the cheddar cheese in 20 second intervals in the microwave, stir carefully to ensure it is melting evenly. It is done when it is completely melted and slightly bubbling on the outside.

3. Mix together all the ingredients while the cheddar is still hot, this will be your dough.

4. Spread the dough out in a flat and even sheet, make sure it is not too thick, you have 37 sausages to cover after all.

5. Preheat your oven to 400F and put the dough in the refrigerator for 15 to 20 minutes to let it harden up a bit.

6. Once it is cold, slice the dough into strips, a pizza cutter is perfect for this, and wrap them around the sausages. Put them in the oven and bake them for 13 to 15 minutes, before you remove them, broil them for an additional one or two minutes.

7.

8. These make a great lunch because they can be reheated once you get to work. You can eat them with a sugar-free ketchup or mustard if you choose. In addition to making a convenient lunch, these also make the perfect snack to bring to a party. When you go to gatherings or parties you might find that there is a lack of ketogenic snacks. Unless otherwise specified, it is safe to assume that you might be faced with a table full of foods you can't eat. The easy solution is to bring your own, these are perfect for that.

9.

10.

11.

12.

13.

14. Tuna Melt Balls with Avocado

15. 10 ounce canned tuna, drained

16. 1 avocado

17. 1/3 cup almond flour

18. ¼ cup mayonnaise, read the label to check for added sugars

19. ¼ cup parmesan cheese

20. ¼ teaspoon onion powder

21. ½ teaspoon garlic powder

22. Salt and pepper to taste

23. ½ coconut oil for frying, approximately a ¼ cup will be absorbed

24.

1. Drain the tuna and put it a bowl that is large enough to hold all of the ingredients.

2. Add the parmesan cheese, spices, and mayonnaise to the tuna and mix it together until evenly coated.

3. Slice your avocado in half and carefully take out the pit, cube the inside. If you have a way that you prefer to cut avocados, feel free to do what makes you comfortable, just make sure the pieces are in small cubes.

4. Add the avocado in with the rest of the mixture, but fold it in slowly, try not to mash it too much, you want pieces to remain.
5. Roll the mixture into balls, about the size of traditional meat balls. Then roll them in the almond flour, make sure they are evenly coated.
6. Put the coconut oil in a pan on medium heat, when it is hot add the tuna balls and fry them until they are brown and crisp on the outside. Make sure you are turning them to ensure each side is cooked properly.
7. Now, simply remove from the pan and serve.
8.
9. These are a great ketogenic version of a tuna melt, you get the creamy center and the added crunch of the outside. Granted, they are not going to be as crunchy when they are reheated, but they are still delicious and easy to take to work with you.
10.
11.
12.
13.

14.

15.

16. Pizza Frittata

17. 9 ounce bag frozen spinach

18. 12 eggs

19. 1 ounce pepperoni

20. 1 teaspoon minced garlic

21. 5 ounce mozzarella cheese

22. ½ cup parmesan cheese

23. ½ cup fresh ricotta cheese

24. 4 tablespoons olive oil

25. ¼ teaspoon nutmeg

26. Salt and pepper to taste

27. Iron skillet or glass container

28.

1. Microwave the frozen spinach for three to four minutes, you don't want to be hot, just defrosted. Then squeeze the spinach with your hands to remove as much water as you can and then set it aside.

2. Preheat your oven to 375F and while it is getting hot, mix together the olive oil, eggs, and spices. Stir or whisk this together until everything is combined.

3. Break the spinach up into small pieces and toss it in the mixture. Next, add the parmesan and ricotta cheeses and mix everything together until it is well combined.
4. Pour your mixture into the skillet and then cover with the mozzarella, place the pepperoni on top just like you would a traditional pizza.
5. Put in the oven and bake for 30 minutes if you are using the cast iron skillet, add an additional 10 to 15 minutes if it is glass. You might need to adjust the baking time depending on the thickness of the frittata, but you will know when it is done when it is slightly browned and firm.
6. Then, just slice and serve.
7.
8. This a perfect lunch to make at the beginning of the week, that will provide enough servings to last the entire week. It is easy to bring to work and once you are there, you can simply heat it up.
9.
10.
11.

12.

13.

14.

15. Chicken and BBQ Soup

16. Base

17. 2 teaspoons chili seasoning

18. 3 chicken thighs

19. 1 ½ cups chicken broth

20. 2 tablespoons of olive oil or chicken fat

21. 1 ½ cups of beef broth

22. Salt and pepper to taste

23.

24. Sauce

25. 1 tablespoon hot sauce

26. ¼ cup reduced sugar ketchup

27. 2 tablespoons Dijon mustard

28. ¼ cup tomato paste

29. 1 teaspoon Worcestershire sauce

30. 2 1.2 teaspoon liquid smoke

31. 1 tablespoon soy sauce

32. 1 teaspoon onion powder

33. 1 teaspoon red chili flakes

34. 1 teaspoon chili powder

35. 1 teaspoon cumin

36. ¼ cup butter

37. 1 ½ teaspoons garlic powder

38. Crock pot or slow cooker

39.

1. Preheat the oven to 400F and remove the bones from the chicken thighs and keep the bones. Season the chicken with some of the chili seasoning and put on a baking tray that is lined with foil.

2. Place the chicken in the oven and bake for 50 minutes.

3. While the chicken is in the oven, grab a pot and add the chicken fat or olive oil, heat this on medium high heat and when it is hot put the chicken bones into the oil and cook them for five minutes. Next, add the broth and season with salt and pepper to taste.

4. When the chicken is done baking, take them out and remove the skins and set aside. Pour the fat from the baked chicken into the broth, stirring occasionally.

5. Now you are going to BBQ sauce by combining all of the ingredients listed above. Then add it to the large pot and stir everything together.

Let the mixture simmer for about 20 to 30 minutes.

6. After it has had time to simmer, use an immersion blender, this will emulsify the liquids and fats together. Shred the chicken and put it in the soup, you can also add bell pepper or spring onions during this step if you choose to and simmer for another 10 to 20 minutes.

7. After it has had time to thicken up, you can now serve it up. You can garnish it with a little cheddar cheese, onions, or some diced up green peppers. The crispy chicken you set aside should also be served on the side as well, it makes a great texture addition to the meal.

8.

9. This is a great lunch option because you can put individual servings in plastic containers and either refrigerate or freeze them for later use. Then when you need a quick lunch on the go, grab the container, throw it your lunch box and be on your way. If that works better for you, than you should really consider utilizing more recipes

like these.

10.

11.

12.

13.

14. **Grilled Cheese Keto Style**

15. 'Bread'

16. 2 tablespoons almond flour

17. 2 eggs

18. 1 ½ tablespoons psyllium husk powder

19. 2 tablespoons soft butter

20. ½ teaspoon baking powder

21.

22. Extras

23. 1 tablespoon butter, soft

24. 2 ounces of white or traditional cheddar

25.

1. Combine the butter, almond flour, baking powder, and psyllium husk in a small bowl.

2. Stir this mixture together as much as you can, it will take the form of a very thick dough.

3. Add the 2 eggs and mix it together, you want your dough to be thick, so it seems too thin,

keep mixing it together, as this will help thicken it up. This can take a full minute or more so be patient.

4. Scoop half the dough out into a square container roughly the size of a slice of bread, or the bottom a bowl to create bun, try to make sure it is spread evenly. You can also use a slightly larger container and cut in half later, if that is what you choose to do, use all the batter. Microwave this for a 90 to 100 seconds. Some might take a little longer to cook thoroughly so check it and it if it still too soft, microwave it for a little longer.

5. Gently remove it from the container by turning it upside down and tapping on the bottom of the container. If you used all of your batter you can cut it in half, if you need to repeat the process to create the other slice of bread, then do so.

6. Place the cheese in between the slices of bread.

7. In a pan set on medium heat add the butter and when it is hot add the sandwich. The

bread will absorb the butter creating that delicious crisp, once it is golden brown, flip and cook the other side until golden brown.

8. Lastly, it is time to eat! A small side salad makes the perfect addition to this gooey, cheesy dish.

9.

10. This is a great comfort food and probably one of the things that you will find yourself craving rather frequently. Again, just because you are on the ketogenic diet does not mean you have to give up everything you love, you just need to learn to make it in new and different ways that won't compromise ketosis.

11.

12. Remember, this is a mix and match meal plan, you do not have to eat all the meals, but do try to keep an open mind. There is no lack of variety when it comes to the ketogenic diet, as a matter of fact, you can still have many of the foods you crave, they will just have a bit of a twist added to them. Whether or not you choose to make your lunches for the whole week or that day is up to you, but you do have

the option. Keep in mind, this will get much easier the more you practice. In the beginning, the key is planning and sticking to it. If you need to create a weekly menu to keep you on track, then do it, there is nothing wrong with it. This is your diet and you have the right to do what works for you.

13.
14.
15.
16.
17.
18.
19.
20.

21.

22. Chapter 5

23. Ketogenic Dinners

24.

25. When it comes to dinners you can be a bit more creative because there isn't typically the need to grab it and go. Most people have more

time to cook a dinner and not have to worry about making enough for a full week or whether or not it will travel well. Just like with the other recipes, you are going to choose your ingredients and keep track of the net carbohydrates you are consuming and since this is the last meal of the day, you will have a good idea of how many net carbohydrates you have let to devote to your dinner.

26.

27. If you have a big dinner planned that you will use up more of your net carbohydrates than usual, make sure to limit your other meals and snacks throughout the day to give yourself the surplus you need for the special dinner. Try not to make this a habit, but everyone has some type of special occasion that requires a more elaborate dinner and this is still possible on the ketogenic diet, it just takes some extra planning. Here is a list of dinner recipes that are perfect for a ketogenic beginner.

28.

29. Chicken with Creamy Greens

30. 1 cup chicken stock

31. 1 pound boneless chicken thighs, with skin

still on

32. 1 cup cream

33. 2 cups dark leafy greens

34. 2 tablespoons coconut oil

35. 2 tablespoons coconut flour

36. 2 tablespoons melted butter

37. 1 teaspoon Italian herbs

38. Salt and pepper to taste

39.

1. In a skillet set on medium high heat add the coconut oil. While this is getting hot, season the chicken with the salt and pepper, make sure to do both sides. When the oil is hot enough, brown the chicken on both sides

2. Continue to fry the chicken until it is crispy and cooked thoroughly. When you are cooking the chicken, you should also start making your sauce.

3. In a sauce pan melt the butter, when it stops sizzling, this means do not let it get brown, only melted, add the coconut flour and begin to whisk it together. Continue to whisk until it forms a thick paste.

4. Add the cream and increase the heat to bring it to a boil, continue to whisk. It will begin to thicken again and when it does, add the Italian herbs.

5. When your chicken is done frying, remove them from the stove and take out the thighs and set them aside.

6. Add the chicken stock into the skillet that just had the chicken in it and deglaze the skillet, slowly add the cream sauce and whisk. Slowly stir the greens into the sauce so they become evenly coated with the sauce.

7. Place the chicken on top of the greens and remove from the stove. You can now serve the meal, when dividing, it makes four servings.

8.

9.

10.

11.

12.

13.

14.

15.

16. Walnut Crusted Salmon

17. 2 tablespoons sugar-free maple syrup

18. 2, 3 ounce salmon fillets

19. ½ cup walnuts

20. 1 tablespoon olive oil

21. ¼ teaspoon dill

22. ½ tablespoon Dijon mustard

23. Salt and pepper to taste

24.

1. Preheat oven to 350F.

2. Put all the walnuts in a food processor with the spices, mustard, and maple syrup. Blend this together until the consistency is very paste like.

3. In a skillet or pan heat up the olive oil until it is very hot, while this is happening dry both sides of the salmon, make sure to a do a good job. When the pan is very hot place the salmon in the pan skin down. Allow it to sear for three minutes.

4. While it searing, spoon the walnut mixture onto the fillets.

5. When they have finished being seared, place them on a pan or foil and place them in the oven to bake for around 8 minutes.

6. This is typically served on a bed of fresh spinach, but if you prefer other leafy greens, the choice is yours.

7.

8. This is a quick and delicious dinner that will leave you feeling satisfied.

9.

10.

11.

12.

13.

14.

15.

16.

17.

18.

19.

20.

21.

22.

23. Crispy Baked Chicken Wings

24. 3 pounds of wings

25. 1 teaspoon baking soda

26. ¼ cup of butter

27. 1 tablespoon salt

28. 2 teaspoons of baking powder

29.

1. In a large plastic bag, dump in the salt, baking powder, baking soda, and all of the chicken wings.

2. Then shake the bag until all of the wings are coated in the mixture, try to make sure it is as even as possible.

3. Put all of the wings on a wire rack and leave in the refrigerator overnight, this will help them dry out which breaks the peptide bonds in the proteins.

4. The next day, preheat your oven to 450F and place the wings in the top middle rack, bake these for 20 minutes.

5. After the first 20 minutes, flip each wing over and bake for an additional 15 minutes or until they are as crispy as you like the,

6. To make a quick buffalo sauce mix together butter and hot sauce and toss them in this to make ketogenic buffalo wings. Enjoy!

7.

8. This is a great dinner for when you have been

watching your friends get their favorite wings from the local spot. When the craving for this type of comfort food hits you, now you can also enjoy them as well.

9.

10.

11.

12.

13.

14.

15.

16.

17.

18.

19.

20.

21.

22.

23.

24.

25.

26. Stuffed Poblanos

27.

28. 1 tablespoon bacon fat

29. 1 pound ground pork
30. ½ onion
31. 4 poblano peppers
32. 7 baby bella mushrooms
33. 1 teaspoon cumin
34. 1 vine tomato
35. 1 teaspoon chili powder
36. ¼ cup chopped cilantro
37. Salt and pepper to taste
38.

1. Rinse and prep all the vegetables, you want to mince garlic, slice the mushrooms and onions, and dice the tomatoes. If your cilantro is not already chopped, do this as well.

2. Set your oven to broil, while this is heating up, place the poblanos on a cookie sheet and put them in the oven when it is hot. Broil them for around 8 to 10 minutes, make sure to move them around every two minutes, you want consistent marks over the entire pepper. Then preheat your oven to 350F.

3. Using a paper towel or gloves to cover your fingers, carefully pull the skin from the peppers. Also, set the skin aside.

4. In a pan that is set on medium high-heat, begin to cook the pork, this is also where you add the bacon fat. Season with salt and pepper, but do not taste it until it has cooked all the way.

5. When it is browned you may now add the chili powder and cumin.

6. In the pan, slide all of the pork to one side and add the garlic and onions to the other side, you want them to be softened.

7. When those have softened add the mushrooms and mix all of it together, add more salt and pepper to suit your palate.

8. When the mixture starts to dry out a little add the tomatoes and cilantro.

9. Make a slice in the poblano pepper from the bottom to the stem and use a spoon or your fingers to remove the seeds. The seeds are spicy, so if you are sensitive to spicy foods, be sure to remove all of them.

10. Carefully fill each pepper with the pork mixture and bake them for around 8 to 10 minutes.

11. Remove them from the oven and they are now ready to serve!

12.

13. These make a unique and fun dinner for what you are craving something simple and spicy. They will probably become a staple in your new diet if you enjoy spicier foods.

14.

15.

16.

17.

18.

19.

20.

21.

22.

23.

24.

25.

26.

27. Coconut Shrimp

28. Shrimp

29. Egg whites from two eggs

30. 1 pound shrimp, deveined and peeled
31. 2 tablespoons coconut flour
32. 1 cup coconut flakes, unsweetened
33.
34. Chili Sauce
35. 1 ½ tablespoon rice wine vinegar
36. 1 diced red chili
37. ½ cup apricot preserves, sugar-free
38. ¼ red pepper flakes
39. 1 tablespoon lime juice
40.

1. If you are using frozen shrimp, make sure you thaw them out first, otherwise, if you bought them fresh peel and devein them if needed. Preheat your oven to 375F.

2. Put the egg whites in a bowl and beat them until soft peaks begin to form, this works best using a hand mixer, or if you are in a pinch, one beater inside a blender also works too.

3. In one bowl put the coconut flakes, in another the coconut flour. Take this time to also grease a cookie sheet.

4. Dip the shrimp in the flour, then dip them in the egg whites, and lastly, the flakes. Arrange

them on the greased cookie sheet and bake them for about 15 minutes, make sure to flip them and broil for 3 to 5 more minutes.

5. To make the sauce simply add all the ingredients into a bowl mix them together. You might have some left over sauce, but it also goes well with chicken!

6.

7. These are a great alternative to chicken nuggets or fried shrimp.

8.

9. Dinners are generally the most fun part of ketogenic cooking because you can really experiment to find what pleases your palate. There are so many different recipes out there already, and you can tweak them so they work for your specific diet needs. Just remember, it might be overwhelming and difficult in the beginning, but you can do it. Just don't give up, let your body adjust and celebrate the small victories like the first pound lost or the first time you didn't have a carb craving all day. This will make the diet more fun and will help keep you motivated.

10.

11.

12. Chapter 6

13. Ketogenic Snacks

14.

15. You are not locked in to only eating three meals a day with no snacking in between. Actually, you can graze a bit throughout the day if that works for you. However, not all snacks are created equal and some are much better than others. Just make sure not to let snacking get out of hand to the point that you are knocked out of ketosis because of it. Don't forget to add in the net carbohydrates from any of the snacks you have eaten throughout the day too, you want an authentic carbohydrate count and this will help make sure it is correct.

16.

17. The best kind of snacks are the ones that you do not have to spend time preparing, and even

though the ketogenic diet is best when you cook at home, there are some things that you can still just grab.

18. Ketogenic Snacks

19. Beef, pork, or chicken jerky

20.

21. String Cheese

22. Seeds, sunflower, pumpkin, and chia

23. Pork rinds, just make sure to read the label, you can even dip them in ketogenic friendly dips such as Ranch or Bleu Cheese dressings.

24.

25. Nut Butters, almond, coconut, and sunflower

26.

27. Sugar-free jello

28.

29. Cocoa nibs, this is the perfect alternative to a chocolate bar

30.

31. In the beginning you might find yourself losing energy or getting hungry at weird times of the day, remember your body is learning to run on something new. So, this is completely normal. These snacks are easy to keep on hand and require no preparation. Just make

sure to add them into your daily carbohydrate intake and they should help you during your transition to a low carbohydrate lifestyle.

32.

33. It probably seems like this diet is overwhelming, but as soon as you get through the first couple of weeks and see the results, you will understand how beneficial it can really be. It will be difficult in the beginning, but you can and should stick it out. You will be proud of yourself in the end. So many people just like you have lost weight and enjoyed healthier lifestyles because of this diet. You don't want to let them reap all the benefits. So, don't let you, hold you back. The secret is finding what works for you and sticking to it, everyone works at their own pace and you are no exception. No matter how badly you might want to compare yourself to others, don't do it. Let your body go at the pace it is meant to, you will learn to know when it is okay to push yourself and when you have truly met your limits, but you won't know either of these until you dedicate yourself and actually try.

34.

35. Conclusion

36.

37. Thank for making it through to the end of *Ketogenic Diet for Beginners: Simple and Fun 3 Weeks Diet Plan for the Smart*, let's hope it was informative and able to provide you with all of the tools you need to achieve your goals whatever it may be.

38. The next step is to start making your meal plans and figuring out how to make the diet work the best for you.

39.

40. **VIP Subscriber List**

41. Hi Dear Reader, this is Diana! If you like my book and you want to receive the latest tips and tricks on cooking, weight-loss, cookbook recipes and more, do subscribe to my mailing list in the link here! I will then be able to send you the most up-to-date information about my upcoming books and promotions as well!

42.

43. **BOOK TWO**

44.

45. THE ULTIMATE WHOLEFOODS COOKBOOK

46.

47. *30 Days To A New You, Health, And*

Body

48.

49.

50. DIANA WATSON

53. Table of Contents

68.

69. Introduction

70.

71. Congratulations on purchasing your personal copy of *The Ultimate Whole Foods Cookbook.* Thank you so much for doing so!

72. The following chapters in this cookbook will cover the basics of what the Whole30 Diet is all about and how you can successfully incorporate it into your everyday lifestyle! While there are many other Whole30 Diet cookbooks on the market, this one covers the absolute basics that you will need to begin your trek down a healthier lane TODAY. This book also contains some of the best recipes from the World Wide Wed, incorporated with recipes that my family, friends and I have tried and enjoyed!

73. You will discover how important is it to be able to eat healthier on YOUR terms and how

this ultimately leads to success in achieving your weight loss goals and assisting in leading a much healthier lifestyle, all while not having to sacrifice delicious tastes!

74. Eating in regards to the Whole Foods Diet is not about eating only certain ingredients like some of those other pesky diet fads, but rather eating less of the food groups that are not so good for our bodies. Our bodies are our temple, so why not fuel it with the best edibles that we can possibly consume? It is a no-brainer!

75. There are plenty of books on this the Whole30 Diet on the market, thanks again for choosing this one! Every effort was made to ensure it is full of as much useful information as possible. Please enjoy!

76.
77.
78.
79.

80.
81.
82.
83.
84.
85.
86.
87.

88. The Basics of the Whole30 Diet
89.
90. Congratulations! If you are reading the first chapter of this book, that means you have decided to take a crucial step in creating a healthier life for yourself and that decision alone is no easy feat! This chapter is all about what the Whole30 diet is, along with what and what not to consume during the course of these vital 30 days. If you have decided to give this diet a try, then you need to be aware that you must be truly committed to wanting to make a change for yourself, as this diet will be asking you to dedicate your time and will-power to sticking directly to the rules of this program.

91. The Whole30 diet is quite the rage nowadays and it is likely that you have heard about it via social media or friends and family. It has also been commonly referred to as more of an

"anti-diet" rather than a regular diet fad, for it is better described as a lifestyle change. The diet itself was designed to be a learning process that you could take along with you for the rest of your life after the initial 30 days. To be able to truly fuel your body in better ways, one must be knowledgeable of how certain edibles affect you. The Whole30 Diet is a perfect blend of the Paleo Diet along with the process of elimination that targets getting rid of foods that are responsible for inflammation within the body.

92. The Whole30 Diet takes crap from no one and says that there is no such thing as "slipping up" when it comes to cheating while on it. Once you know which foods to keep yourself from consuming, you must keep them out of your life as you retrain your body not to crave them. That is the entire goal of this 30-day

diet: to identify the bad foods and 100% eliminate them from your diet for hopefully, well, forever. This means you must be prepared to make this type of lifestyle change, for it won't be the easiest thing to rid yourself of your everyday bowl of ice cream or other bad eating habits.

93. The good news? There are plenty of recipes out there that you can consume that are delicious enough to keep you from thinking about those edibles you crave every day. The best place to start is within the other chapters of this book when searching for recipes to incorporate into your life.

94.

95.

96. The Whole30 Day Rules

97. Do's

- **Consume real foods**
  - Eat foods such as eggs, seafood, and meat in moderated proportions.
  - Lots of vegetables
  - Portioned fruits
  - Lots of seasonings, spices, herbs, and natural fats
  - Foods with fewer ingredients are far better. This means that they are more than likely less processed than foods with long ingredient lists.
  - Look for foods that contain ingredients you can pronounce
  - **Don'ts: To be avoided for 30 days**
- **No junk foods, baked good or other goodies with "approved" components**

- Any of these types of edibles, even those with ingredients that are "technically" within Whole30 limitations, disregard the entire point of going on this diet, to begin with. It will compromise your potential results.

- **No sulfites, MSG or carrageenan**

- **No dairy**

- Includes sheep, goat and cow milk

- Includes frozen yogurt, ice cream, sour cream, yogurt, kefir, cheese, cream, and milk

- **No legumes**

- Includes beans of ALL kinds

- Includes peanut butter and other such butters

- Includes soy in ALL forms

- **No grains**

- Includes:

- Sprouted grains, sorghum, bulgur, millet, rice, corn, oats, barley, rye, and wheat

- ALL gluten-free cereals: quinoa, buckwheat, etc

- Also includes processes in which the above are added into foods. *Important to read food labels*.

- **No alcohol**

- **No sugar**

  o This includes both real and artificial kinds of sugar

- **Do not step on the scale or take measurements for entire 30 days**

  o This diet is not only about weight loss, but curbing your bad eating habits which will lead to benefits that have the potential to last a lifetime.

  o **Exceptions – Allowed during the**

course of the Whole30

- **Salt**
- **Coconut aminos**
- **Vinegar**
- **Particular legumes**

  ○ Snow and sugar snap peas and green beans are allowed. These foods are pods rather than beans.

- **Fruit juices**
- **Clarified butter or ghee**
- **You have ONE job – Let Whole30 Do the Rest**
- Your job while on the course of this diet is to stay away from food that is off limits and fulfill your stomach with the edibles that are allowed. There is no need for the hassle of constantly weighing yourself. These is no need to write down weekly measurements. There is no reason to count all those calories that you

consume. There are no requirements to waste your hard earned money on buying organic products. If you learn how to truly reside closely to the Whole30 rules for the entirety of 30 consecutive days, the diet will provide you with spectacular results! The remainder of this book is filled with delectable recipes to fulfill your cravings and keep you on the right track while on the Whole30 Diet.

-
-
-
-
-
-
-

Whole30 Breakfast Recipes

Zucchini Noodle Breakfast Bowl

What's in it:

- Salt and pepper
- 2 tbsp. green onion
- 2 eggs
- 2 sweet potatoes
- 1-2 cloves of garlic
- 2 tbsp. water
- ¼ c. olive oil
- ½ avocado
- 1-2 zucchinis

How it's made:

- Skin sweet potatoes and proceed to cut them into bite sized pieces. In a skillet, heat olive oil over medium heat and cook potatoes, ensuring to stir occasionally.
- Take zucchini, cut off ends and then put through a spiralizer and set to the side.
- Avocado cream: Put water, 2 tablespoons olive oil, garlic and avocado into food processor and pulse, adding more olive oil if needed
- Pour avocado cream over zucchini noodles and toss until coated. Take cooked and lightly browned potatoes and pour over noodles
- Utilizing the skillet you cooked potatoes in, cook your eggs until they are done to your liking and put over top of noodles.
- Plate with green onion, using salt and pepper to taste

- **Four-Ingredient Granola Bars**
-
- **What's in it:**
-
- 3 tbsp. water
- ¾ c. dried cranberries
- 2 c. desiccated coconut
- 2 c. walnuts
- 1 c. pitted dates
-
- **How it's made:**
-
- Preheat over to 170 degrees then proceed to toast walnuts. Let cool before putting in a food processor. Add in cranberries, coconut, and dates
- Mix until well combined and crumbly
- Add water one tablespoon at a time, creating a mixture sticky in texture that is able to hold together
- Line cling wrap in a baking dish, preferably square and then press the mixture inside it
- Place inside fridge for a couple to few hours
- Sprinkle with coconut and cut into bars
-

Whole30 Lunch Recipes

Sausage and Kale Sauté

What's in it:

- ½ of a chopped red bell pepper
- 1 diced onion
- 1 bunch kale
- 1 pound sausage

How it's made:

- In a large pan, brown sausage
- Add onion in pan and cook until they are soft and translucent in color
- Remove kale spine and chop into bite sized pieces
- Add kale to pan. Cook and stir until kale leaves are bright green in color and is a texture you prefer
- Remove kale and sausage mixture from the pan and stir in red pepper. Serve while warm

Turkey Plantain Nachos

What's in it:

- 2 c. lettuce, shredded
- 1 6 oz. bag plantain chips
- 2 tbsp. taco seasoning
- 1 pound of lean ground turkey
- Other toppings: guacamole, salsa, tomatoes, peppers, onions, etc.

- **How it's made:**
-
- Brown turkey in a skillet
- While turkey is cooking, prepare toppings
- Once turkey is cooked, add taco seasoning and stir until combined.
- Place plantain chips on bottom, then lettuce, turkey, and other toppings in an order that your taste buds prefer. Enjoy!
-
-
-
-
-
-
-
-
-
-
-
-

Whole30 Dinner Recipes

Roasted Lemon Chicken with Potatoes

What's in it:

- ½ tsp. salt and pepper
- ½ tsp. red pepper flakes
- 1 tbsp. rosemary
- 2 cloves garlic
- 1/3 c. olive oil
- 2 lemons, sliced and juiced
- ½ onion
- 1 pound baby red potatoes
- 8-10 pieces of chicken with skin on and bone in

How it's made:

- Ensure oven is preheated to 400 degrees
- Prime 1 13x9 glass baking dish with cooking spray. Place pieces of chicken with skin side up with potatoes, cut up onion and lemon slices, ensuring that all ingredients are even in pan
- Mix together lemon juice, red pepper flakes, salt, pepper, rosemary and garlic in a small bowl

- Pour this mixture over the chicken, tossing to ensure even coating
- Sprinkle with pepper and salt
- Bake chicken, uncover, for an hour or until cooked
-
- **Tomato Basil Beef Goulash with Eggplant**
-
- **What's in it:**
-
- ¾ c. coconut cream
- 2 tbsp. tomato paste
- 2 tsp. salt
- 1/3 c. basil
- 1 14 oz. can diced tomatoes
- 1 eggplant
- 1 pound ground beef
- 4 garlic gloves
- 2 shallots
- 2 tbsp. olive oil
-
- **How it's made:**
-
- In a large saucepan, heat olive oil, then add garlic and shallots. Sauté until fragrant
- Add in beef and cook until browned
- In another pan, heat more olive oil and pour in eggplant, cooking until soft
- Once beef is cooked, drain grease and add tomatoes, salt, and basil. Stir until well-combined, then add in coconut cream, eggplant and tomato paste
- Serve with garnish and more basil
-
-
-

●

Whole30 Dessert Recipes

Banana, Cinnamon, and Nutmeg Ice Cream

What's in it:

- Cinnamon and nutmeg
- ½ c. coconut milk
- 1 c. frozen bananas

How it's made:

Place all ingredients into a blender until combined. If too thick, add more coconut milk.
Enjoy!

Coconut Almond Butter Truffles

What's in it:

- ¼ tsp. almond extract
- Pinch of salt
- 2 tbsp. almond butter
- ¼ c. coconut butter

Optional:

- ½ tbsp. coconut oil
- 1 tsp. unsweetened cocoa powder

How it's made:

- In a small bowl, mix together almond butter and coconut and warm in microwave until melted, stirring until smooth in texture
- Add almond extract and salt and stir
- Freeze for around 10 minutes until hardened
- After freezing, roll into balls and then return back to freezing
- In a small bowl, melt coconut oil and stir in cocoa powder until combined. Dip balls into mixture of chocolate and let chocolate set. Re-dip for thicker coating and let sit until set.
- Keep in fridge if all of them aren't eaten at once!
-
- **Raw Brownie Bites**
-
- **What's in it:**
-
- 1/3 c. unsweetened cocoa powder
- 1 tsp. vanilla
- 1 c. pitted dates
- Pinch of salt
- 1 ½ c. walnuts
-
- **How it's made:**
-
- In a food processor, finely grind walnuts and salt
- Add cocoa powder, vanilla and dates into food processor. Mix until everything is combined. Add water a little at a time until you have a mixture that sticks together
- Put mixture into a bowl. Use hands and form small balls. Store in container within the fridge for up to one week.
-

-
-
-
-
-
-
-
-
-
-
-
-
-
-

-
- Conclusion
-
- Thank for making it through to the end of *30 Day Whole Foods Cookbook: The Only 30 Days You Ever Need to Great Health.* I hope that you found the contents of this book is everything you needed to get started on incorporating the Whole30 Diet directly into your lifestyle as soon as possible!

- The contents of this cookbook should have provided you with all the necessary tools to achieve your goals to a better diet plan. You have within your hands the perfect vessel to lead you to a path of healthier eating, with the perfect amount of meals and other recipes to get you started on the right foot!

- Isn't it about time that you took the initiative to feel better about yourself inside AND out? Wouldn't it be an amazing feeling to have the energy to do all the things you love every day?

Isn't it about time that you took the initiative to healthier living today rather than waiting until tomorrow?

- The next step is to put the rules of the Whole30 Diet to work for you, starting with making the delicious recipes that are included in the contents of this book! All these recipes go great with your other favorite eats, as well as paired with other recipes that are within the chapters of this cookbook!

- I hope that the contents of this cookbook will help you gain the confidence to start incorporating healthier lifestyle habits within your everyday life today!

-
-
-

-

-

BOOK THREE

KETOGENIC DIET

Better Energy, Performance, and Natural Fuel to Good Health for the Smart

• DIANA WATSON

- Copyright © 2017 DIANA WATSON
  -

-
-
-
-
-
-
-

• Table of Contents

-
- Introduction
- Chapter 1: The Keto Plan & How it WorksC
- Chapter 2: 14-Day Plan
- Chapter 3: Additional Breakfast Recipes
- Chapter 4: Additional Lunch & Dinner Recipes
- Chapter 5: Snacks and Desserts for the Diet Plan
- Conclusion

- <u>Index</u>

VIP Subscriber List

Hi Dear Reader, this is Diana! If you like my book and you want to receive the latest tips and tricks on cooking, weight-loss, cookbook recipes and more, do subscribe to my mailing list in the link here! I will then be able to send you the most up-to-date information about my upcoming books and promotions as well! Thank you for supporting my work and happy reading!

Subscriber Form

http://bit.do/dianawatson

Introduction

Congratulations on purchasing the *Ketogenic Diet: Better Energy, Performance, and Natural Fuel to Good Health for the Smart*, and thank you for doing so.

The following chapters will discuss many different ways you can eat healthier using a high-fat diet that remains low in carbohydrates. An extensive amount of research has been provided to prove how this type of plan can improve your health and help you lose the unwanted pounds.

It works using the process of ketosis which will be briefly explained.

There are plenty of books on this subject on the market, thanks again for choosing this one! Every effort was made to ensure it is full of as much useful information as possible; please enjoy!

Chapter 1: The Keto Plan & How it Works

You will soon understand how you can eat most of the foods you always enjoy. You will be able to make some substitutes to get going which are described within this chapter.

Happy Discovery!

Several Types of Keto Diet Plans

- *Plan 1*: You can choose from the standard ketogenic diet (SKD) which consists of high-fat, moderate protein, and is extremely low in carbs.

- *Plan 2*: The cyclical ketogenic diet or CKD is created with 5-keto days trailed by two high-carb days.

- *Plan 3*: The targeted keto diet, which is also called TKD, will provide you with a plan to add carbs to the diet during the times when you are working out.

- *Plan 4*: The high-protein ketogenic diet is very

similar to the standard keto plan in all aspects except that it has more protein.

- However, let's not get too far ahead of the plan. You need to focus on the first 30 days! The long process to explain each of these types would take another entire book!

- **Health Benefits from a Ketogenic Diet Plan**

- These are just a few of the ways you can benefit from remaining on the diet plan. It's hard to believe a diet plan can remedy so many health issues.

- *Acne*: Your insulin levels are lowered by consuming less sugar and eating less processed foods. The acne will begin to clear up as you continue with the plan.

- *Alzheimer's disease*: The symptoms and progression will be slowed.

- *Lowered Blood Pressure*: While using the keto plan; you are experiencing reduced intake of carbs which will reduce your blood pressure levels. It is recommended to seek advice from your regular doctor to see if it is possible to reduce some of your medication while you are on the keto diet. You may also have some dizziness when you first begin the plan which is one of the first indications that the plan is working. The result is a lack of carbohydrates.

- *Cancer*: Slow tumor growths and several other types of cancer have shown improvement with the keto plan.

- *Diabetes and Pre-diabetes*: The main link to pre-diabetes is excess body fat which is removed which is proven by research that insulin sensitivity was improved by as much as 70%.

- *Epilepsy*: Children's research studies have proven the diet works in the reduction of seizure activity.

- *Gum Disease*: The sugar you consume influences the pH balance in your mouth. If you have issues before you begin the plan; you should begin to see a remarkable improvement within approximately three months.

- *Obesity*: When the ketogenic diet plan is followed—the weight will dissolve.

- *Stiffness and Joint Pain*: It is important to continue with the elimination of any grain-based foods. It is believed that the grains are one of the largest factors which cause the pain. Just remember "no grain—no pain."

- *Thinking is Improved*: You might be a bit foggy-minded when you first begin the plan since you will be consuming high-fat foods. After all, your brain is about 60% fat by weight; your thinking skills should improve with the intake of the fatty foods indicated with the keto diet.

- **The Elements of Ketosis**

- Ketosis is used to help your burn body fat and drop extra pounds. Proteins will fuel your body to burn the fat—therefore—the ketosis will maintain your muscles and make you less hungry.

- Your body will remain healthy and work as it should. If you don't consume enough carbs from your food; your cells will begin to burn fat for the necessary energy instead. Your body will switch over to ketosis for its energy source as your cut back on your calories and carbs.

- Two elements that occur when your body doesn't need the glucose:

- *Lipogenesis*: If there is a sufficient supply of glycogen in your liver and muscles, any excess is converted to fat and stored.

- *Glycogenesis:* The excess of glucose converts to glycogen and is stored in the muscles and liver. Research indicates that only about half of your energy used daily can be stored as glycogen.

- As a result, your body will have no more food—similar to when you are sleeping—your body burns the fat and creates ketones. These ketones break down the fats, which generate fatty acids, and burn-off in the liver through beta-oxidation.

- Simply stated, when you no longer have a supply of glycogen or glucose, ketosis begins and will use the consumed/stored fat as energy.

- The Internet provides you with a keto

calculator to use at http://keto-calculator.ankerl.com/. You can check your levels when you want to know what essentials your body needs during your diet plan or after. All you need to do is document your personal information such as weight and height. The calculator will provide you with the essential math.

- **Weight Loss and Protein**
- Protein needs to be in your plan for these reasons:
- *Protein is a Fat Burner:* Science has proven your body cannot use and burn your fat as energy sources unless you have help from either carbs or protein. The balance of protein must be maintained to preserve your calorie-burning lean muscles.
- *Protein Saves Your Calories:* Protein slows down your digestion process making you feel

more satisfied from the foods you eat. During the first cycle of your diet plan; it is imperative that you feel full, so there is no temptation to cheat on the strategy.

- *Muscle Repair and Growth*: Protein should be increased on days when you are more active. It is essential to have a plan on what your meals will consist of with a balance of carbs, proteins, and calories. The balance is what you are attempting to achieve with a focused plan such as the keto diet.

- **The Role of Calories, Protein, and Carbs**

- Calories are held within your body with the use of the nutrients of protein, fat, and carbs which your body will use for energy.

- **Carbohydrates**

- Your body exchanges one-hundred percent of the carbs into glucose which gives your body an energy boost. About 50% to 60% of your intake of calories is produced by carbs. Carbs stored in your liver as glycogen is released as your body needs it. Glucose is essential for the creation of adenosine triphosphate (ATP) which is an energy molecule. The fuel from glucose is vital for the daily maintenance and activities inside your body. After the liver has reached its maximum capacity for its limits, the excessive carbohydrates turn into fat.

- **Count Those Carbs**
- Before you are totally in gear, you need to start carb counting to make sure you keep your body in perfect 'sync' with the plan. Reading the labels may be a bit nerve-racking in the beginning, but after a while, it will be as you have always done it that way.
- *Remember this Formula*: Total Carbs minus (-) Fiber = Net Carbs
- A rough estimate will include you consuming

between 20 to 30 carbs daily. It is almost a necessity to own a set of food scales to take out the guesswork.

- Keep this information in mind before you make the purchase:
- *The Automatic Shut-Off*: Seek a scale that does not have this option. The result could be you being in the midst of a recipe—move the dish —and the scale could reset; NOT.
- *The Tare Function*: When you set a bowl on the scale, the feature will allow you to reset the scale back to zero (0).
- *Removable Plate*: Keep the germs off of the scale by removing the plate. Be sure it will come off to eliminate the bacterial buildup.
- *Seek a Conversion Button*: You need to know how to convert measurements into grams since not all recipes have them listed. The grams keep the system in complete harmony.

- **Natural Supplements for Ketogenic Dieters**

- *Fermented Foods:* Use items, while on the keto plan such as coconut milk kefir, coconut milk, yogurt, pickles, sauerkraut, and kimchi to help with any digestive issues.

- *Lemon and Lime:* Your blood sugar levels will naturally drop with these citric additions, and signal a boost in your liver function. Use them in green juices, with a salad, or with cooked with meats or veggies. The choices are limitless and assist you with the following:

- Reduces toothache pain

- Boosts your immune system

- Relieves respiratory infections

- Balances pH

- Decreases wrinkles and blemishes

- Reduces fever

- Excellent for weight loss

- Flushes out the unwanted, unhealthy materials
- Blood purifier
- *Apple Cider Vinegar*: Who would believe the benefits you can receive from just one to two tablespoons of vinegar in an 8-ounce glass of water would help the process? You can choose the straight up method and skip the water. These are just a few ways this helps your progress:
- Reduces cholesterol
- Excellent for detoxification
- Helps you to drop the pounds
- Improves your digestion tract
- Helps with sore muscles
- Controls sugar intake/aids in diabetes
- Strengthens your immune system
- A good energy booster
- Balances your inner body system and functions
- *Cinnamon*: Use cinnamon as part of your daily

plan to improve your insulin receptor activity. Just put one-half of a teaspoon of cinnamon into a shake or any type of keto dessert. Many of the keto recipes contain the ingredient.

- *Turmeric*: Dating back to Ayurveda and Chinese medicine the is of this Asian orange herb has been known for its anti-inflammatory compounds. Add it to you smoothies, green drinks, meats, or veggies. These are some of its benefits:

- Prevents Alzheimer's disease

- Weight management

- Relieves arthritis

- Reduces your cholesterol levels

- Helps control diabetes

- Improves your digestion

- **Be Aware of Some Foods and Beverages: Which Ones to Avoid**

- *Agave Nectar*: One teaspoon has 5 grams of carbs versus 4 grams in table sugar.

- *Beans and Legumes*: This group to avoid includes peas, lentils, kidney beans, and chickpeas. If you use them, be sure to count the carbs, protein, and fat content.

- *Cashews and Pistachios*: The high carb content should be monitored for these yummy nuts.

- *Fruits*: Raspberries, blueberries, and cranberries contain high sugar contents. In small portions; you can enjoy some strawberries.

- *Grains and Starches*: Avoid wheat-based items such as cereal, rice, or pasta.

- *Hydrogenated Fats*: Cold-pressed items should be avoided when using vegetable oils such as safflower, olive, soybean, or flax. Coronary heart disease has been linked to these fats

which also include margarine.

- *Tomato-based Products*: Read the labels because most of the tomato products contain sugar. If you use them be sure to account for the sugar content. (The recipes provided have considered this.)

-
-

• Chapter 2: The 14-Day Plan

-

• Day One

- **Breakfast: Keto Scrambled Eggs**

- *Ingredients*

- 3 large eggs

- Fresh ground pepper

- Coarse salt

- 1 tablespoon unsalted butter

- *Instructions*

1. Whisk the eggs in a bowl.

2. Use low heat and place the butter into a skillet.

3. Add the eggs. Continue to stir until well-done, usually 1 ½ to 3 minutes.

4. *Serving Portion:* Fat: 26.3 g; Carbs 1.8 g; Protein: 17.4 g; Calories: 318

5. **Lunch: Tuna Cheese Melt (Low-Carbs)**
6. *Ingredients*

7. 2 Pieces of "Oopsie" bread

8. *Ingredients for the Salad*

9. 1 to 2 Celery stalks

10. 5 1/3 Tablespoons sour cream or mayonnaise

11. 1 Can tuna (in olive oil)

12. 4 Tablespoons chopped dill pickles

13. ½ teaspoon lemon juice

14. Pepper and salt to taste

15. ½ minced clove garlic

16. *Toppings*

17. A pinch of paprika powder or cayenne pepper

18. 3 ½ ounces shredded cheese

19. *Serving Ingredients*

20. Olive oil

21. 1/3 Pound leafy greens

22. *"Oopsie" Bread (makes six to 8)*

23. 3 Eggs

24. A pinch of salt

25. 4 ¼ ounces cream cheese

26. ½ teaspoon baking powder

27. ½ Tablespoon ground psyllium husk powder

28. *Instructions*

1. Preheat the oven to 350ºF. Put parchment paper onto a cookie sheet.

2. Blend all of the salad ingredients.

3. Place the bread slices on the prepared sheet, spread the tuna, and sprinkle the cheese on top of each slice of bread.

4. Sprinkle some cayenne or paprika powder on the sandwich halves and bake in the oven for about 15 minutes.

5. Have some leafy greens with a drizzle of olive oil.

6. *"Oopsie" Bread Instructions*

1. Heat the oven to oven at 300ºF.

2. Begin by separating the egg whites (whites in one bowl and yolks in the other).

3. Whisk the egg whites with the salt until peaks are formed.

4. Combine the cream cheese and egg yolks—add the baking powder and psyllium seed husk (making it more Oopsie type bread).

5. Blend/fold in the whites into the yolk mixture —keeping out the air in the whites of the eggs.

6. Place six or eight 'oopsies' on the paper-lined sheet.

7. Bake in the center oven rack, usually for 25 minutes or until browned.

8. Dinner: Chicken Smothered in Creamy Onion Sauce

9. *Ingredients*

10. 1 whole green/spring onion

11. 2 tablespoons or 1-ounce butter

12. 4 chicken breast halves (skinless—boneless)

13. 8 ounces sour cream

14. ½ teaspoon sea salt

15. *Note*: The chicken should weigh approximately six ounces or 170 g for this recipe.

16. *Instructions*

1. In a large pan, melt the butter on the stovetop using the med-high setting. Lower the heat setting to med-low—put the chicken with the butter—cover and cook about ten more minutes.
2. Chop the onion using just the white and green sections.
3. Flip the breasts—cover and simmer—another 8 or 9 minutes (or until completely done).
4. Combine the onion, and continue cooking the chicken for another one or two minutes.
5. Take it off of the burner, and blend in the salt and sour cream.
6. Let the meal rest and flavors blend for five minutes.
7. Stir well and serve.

8. Day Two

9. Breakfast: Mock Mc Griddle Casserole

10. *Ingredients*

11. 1 pound breakfast sausage

12. ¼ cup flaxseed meal

13. 1 cup almond flour

14. 10 large eggs

15. 6 tablespoons maple syrup

16. 4 ounces cheese

17. 4 tablespoons butter

18. ¼ teaspoon sage

19. ½ teaspoon each: onion & garlic powder

20. *Instructions*

1. **Heat the oven to 350ºF. Use parchment paper to line a 9 x 9-inch casserole dish.**

2. **Using medium heat; start cooking the breakfast sausage on the stove in a skillet.**

3. **Blend all of the dry (the cheese included) ingredients and add the wet ones.**

4. **Add four tablespoons of the syrup and blend well.**

5. After the sausage is crispy brown—blend all of the ingredients; (the fat too).

6. Pour the mixture into the dish and sprinkle the remainder of the syrup on the top.

7. Bake for 45 to 55 minutes. Remove it and let it cool.

8. Yields: Eight Servings
9. *Time Saving Tip*: The casserole should be easy to remove by using the edge of the parchment paper.

10. **Lunch: Brussels Sprouts with Hamburger Gratin**

11. *Ingredients*

12. 1 Pound Ground beef

13. 1 Pound Brussels sprouts

14. ½ Pound diced bacon

15. 4 tablespoons sour cream

16. 1/3 Pound shredded cheese

17. 1- ¾ Ounces butter

18. Pepper and salt to taste

19. 1 tablespoon Italian seasoning

20. Instructions

1. Cut the Brussels sprouts in half.

2. Preheat the oven to 425ºF/220ºC.

3. Saute the Brussels sprouts and bacon in the butter. Flavor with the sour cream and place in a baking pan/dish.

4. Fry the beef and season with pepper and salt; add the herbs and cheese—sprinkling on top of the base layer.

5. Bake on the center rack of the oven for fifteen minutes.

6. Serve with a dollop of mayonnaise and a fresh salad.

7. *Yields:* Four Servings

8.

9. Dinner: Squash and Sausage Casserole

10. Ingredients

11. 1 pound browned sausage

12. 2 large eggs

13. 1 medium zucchini (sliced & cooked)

14. 2 medium summer squash (sliced & cooked)

15. 1 teaspoon salt

16. ½ teaspoon onion powder or ¼ cup dried minced onion

17. 1 cup mayonnaise

18. 1 package sugar substitute (or stevia)

19. ¼ teaspoon pepper

20. 1 ½ cups shredded cheddar cheese (divided)

21. ¼ melted butter

22. *Instructions*

1. Pre-set the oven to 350ºF.

2. Blend each of the ingredients except for one-half of a cup of shredded cheese.

3. Put the ingredients into a lightly greased oblong baking plate.

4. Sprinkle the remainder of cheese on the casserole.

5. Bake until lightly browned for approximately thirty minutes.

6. This casserole will easily serve 12 people with an amazing flavor you won't soon forget!

7. Day Three

8. Breakfast: Can't Beat it Porridge

9. *Ingredients*

10. 1 cups almond or coconut milk

11. 1 pinch salt

12. 1 Tablespoon each:

- Sunflower seeds

- Chia Seeds

- *Instructions*

1. Using a small saucepan on the stovetop, blend each of the components, and bring to a boiling. Lower the burner and cook slowly until the porridge is the consistency you desire

2. Garnish with some butter or milk. You can also add some fresh unsweetened berries or cinnamon.

3. *Yields:* One Serving

4. *Time Saving Tip:* Make it ahead of time using a big glass jar. Fill the jar with the following ingredients and shake them up. Each serving will correspond with three tablespoons for each serving.

5. *These are the ingredients needed for the batch:*

6. 1 Tbsp. cinnamon

7. ½ tsp. salt

8. 1 1/4 cup each:

- Sunflower seeds

- Flaxseeds

- Chia seeds

- **Lunch: Salad From a Jar**

- *Ingredients*

- 1 (4-ounce) rotisserie chicken/smoked salmon/ other protein
- 1 ounce each:
- Cucumber
- Cherry tomatoes
- Leafy greens
- Bell pepper
- 4 tablespoons olive oil or mayonnaise
- ½ Scallion
- *Instructions*

1. Chop or shred the veggies and place the leafy greens to the bottom for a crunch followed by the colorful veggies. (You can also use some cauliflower or broccoli for a change of pace.)

2. Top it off with some of the grilled protein of your choice. You can also use cold cuts, tuna fish, mackerel or boiled eggs.

3. Cheese cubes, seeds, nuts, and olives are also healthy and colorful additions.

4. Add a generous amount of mayonnaise or salad dressing and enjoy!

5. *Yields*: One Serving

6. **Dinner: Ham and Cheese Stromboli**

7. *Ingredients*

8. 1 large egg

9. 1 ¼ cups shredded mozzarella cheese

10. 3 tablespoons coconut flour

11. 4 tablespoons almond flour

12. 4 ounces of ham

13. 1 teaspoon Italian seasoning

14. 3 ½ ounces cheddar cheese

15. *Instructions*

1. Preheat the oven to 400ºF.

2. Melt the mozzarella cheese in the microwave for one minute/alternating at ten-second intervals; stirring until melted.

3. In a mixing bowl, blend the coconut and almond flour with the seasonings.

4. Toss in the mozzarella on the top and work it in.

5. After the cheese has cooled; beat the egg and combine everything

6. On a flat surface; put some parchment paper, and add the mixture.

7. Use a rolling pin or your hands to flatten the mix.

8. Place several diagonal lines using a knife or pizza cutter. (Leave a row of approximately four inches wide in the center.

9. Alternate the layers using the cheddar and ham on the uncut space of dough until you have used all of the filling.

10. Bake for 15 to 20minutes or it is browned.

11. Day Four

12. Breakfast: Frittata with Cheese and Tomatoes

13. Ingredients

14. 6 eggs

15. 2/3 cup soft cheese (ex. Feta 3 ½ ounces or 100 g)

16. ½ medium white onion (1.9 ounces or 55 g)

17. 2/3 cup halved cherry tomatoes

18. 2 tablespoons chopped herbs (ex. basil or chives)

19. 1 tablespoon ghee/butter

20. *Instructions*

1. Heat the oven broiler to 400ºF.

2. Place the onions on a greased, hot iron skillet, and cook with ghee/butter until slightly brown.

3. In a separate container, crack the eggs and add the salt, pepper, or add herbs of your choice. Whisk and add to the onion pan.

4. Cook until the edges begin to get brown. Top with the cheese and tomatoes.

5. Put the pan in the broiler for five to seven minutes or until done.

6. Lunch: Chicken—Broccoli—Zucchini Boats

7. For a variety textures as well as flavors to spice up lunch; this is the one!

8. *Ingredients*

9. 6 ounces shredded chicken

10. 2 tablespoons butter

11. 2 hollowed-out zucchini (10 ounces)

12. 3 ounces shredded cheddar cheese

13. 1 stalk of green onion

14. 1 cup broccoli

15. 2 tablespoons sour cream

16. *Instructions*

1. Heat the oven temperature to 400ºF.

2. Slice the zucchini lengthwise and scoop most of the insides out until you have a shell of approximately ½ to 1 cm. thick.

3. Melt one tablespoon of the butter into each boat, flavor with a dash of pepper and salt, and bake them for around twenty minutes.

4. Shred the chicken, cut the broccoli florets into small pieces, and measure out six ounces of cheese. Blend in with the sour cream.

5. Remove the zucchini shells when done and add the mixture.

6. Sprinkle each of them with the remainder of the cheese.

7. Bake for another ten or fifteen minutes until the cheese is browned and melted.

8. Use a bit of sour cream, mayonnaise, or chopped onion as a garnish.

9. **Dinner: Steak-Lovers Slow-Cooked Chili**

10. *Ingredients for Chili*:

11. 1 cup beef or chicken stock

12. ½ cup sliced leeks

13. 2 ½ pounds (1-inch cubes) steak

14. 2 cups whole tomatoes (canned with juices)

15. 1 tablespoon chili powder

16. ½ tsp. salt

17. 1/8 tsp. ground black pepper

18. ¼ tsp. ground cayenne pepper

19. ½ tsp. cumin

20. *Optional Toppings*

21. 1 teaspoon fresh chopped cilantro

22. 2 tablespoons sour cream

23. ¼ cup shredded cheddar cheese

24. ½ avocado (cubed or sliced)

25. *Instructions*

1. Place all of the items except the topping fixings into the slow cooker.

2. Set the cooker on the high setting for about six hours.

3. *Yields:* Twelve Servings

4. *Serving Portion: 1:* Fat: 26.0 g; Carbs 3.3 g; Protein: 38.4 g; Calories: 321

5. *Servings with Toppings: Serving Portion: 1:* Fat: 41.32 g; Carbs 13.49 g; Protein: 32.47 g; Calories: 540.33

6. Day 5
7. Breakfast: Brownie Muffins

8. Ingredients

9. ½ tsp. salt

10. 1 cup flaxseed meal

11. ¼ cup cocoa powder

12. ½ Tbsp. baking powder

13. 1 Tbsp. cinnamon

14. 2 Tbsp. coconut oil

15. 1 large egg

16. 1 tsp. vanilla extract

17. ¼ cup sugar-free caramel syrup

18.   ½ cup pumpkin puree

19. ¼ cup slivered almonds

20. 1 tsp. apple cider vinegar

21. Instructions

1. Heat the oven temperature at 350ºF.

2. In a deep mixing bowl—combine all of the ingredients—mixing well.

3. Use six paper liners in the muffin tin, and add ¼ cup of the batter to each one.

4. Sprinkle several almonds on the tops, pressing gently.

5. Bake approximately fifteen minutes. It is done when the top is set.

6. *Serving Portion:* 1 muffin (The recipe serves six): Fat: 13.4 g; Carbs 8.2 g; Protein: 7 g; Calories: 183.3

7. **Lunch: Bacon-Avocado-Goat Cheese Salad**

8. *Ingredients*

9. ½ Pound bacon

10. ½ Pound goat cheese

11. 4 ounces walnuts

12. 2 avocados

13. 4 ounces arugula lettuce

14. *Ingredients for the Dressing*

15. 7 ½ tablespoons mayonnaise

16. Juice of ½ of a lemon

17. 2 tablespoons heavy whipping cream

18. 7 ½ tablespoons olive oil

19. *Instructions*

1. Preheat the oven temperature to 400ºF/200ºC.

2. Prepare a baking dish with some parchment paper.

3. Slice the goat cheese into ½-inch round slices and put in the baking dish. Place on the upper rack of the oven.

4. Pan-fry the bacon until crunchy.

5. Cut the avocados and place on top of a bed of lettuce, add the bacon, cheese, and nuts to the top of your creation.

6. Make the dressing using a stick blender. Sprinkle in a dash of pepper, salt, or a few fresh herbs.

7. *Yields*: Four Servings

8. **Dinner: Tenderloin Stuffed Keto Style**

9. *Ingredients*

10. 2 pounds pork tenderloin or venison

11. ½ cup feta cheese

12. ½ cup gorgonzola cheese

13. 1 teaspoon chopped onion

14. 2 tablespoons crushed almonds

15. 2 garlic cloves, minced

16. ½ teaspoon each: fresh ground black pepper

   and sea salt

17. Instructions

1. Preheat the grill.

2. Form a pocket in the tenderloin.

3. Mix the cheeses, almonds, garlic, and onions.

4. Stuff the pocket, and seal using a skewer.

5. Grill until its desired doneness.

6. *Yields:* Eight Servings

7. *Serving Portion: 1:* Fat: 6.2 g; Carbs 2.9 g;

   Protein: 28.8 g; Calories: 194

8. Day 6
9. Breakfast: Sausage—Feta—Spinach

   Omelet

10. *Ingredients*

11. ½ tablespoon extra-virgin olive oil

12. 2 sausage links

13. 3 large eggs

14. ¼ cup Half & Half

15. 1 cup spinach

16. 1 tablespoon feta cheese

17. *Note:* You will need two skillets for this yummy omelet!

18. *Instructions*

1. Use medium heat for both pans, and pour olive oil in one of the two.

2. In a small dish, use the Half & Half and mix with the eggs—add the seasonings—and scramble.

3. In the clean pan, cook the sausage.

4. Sauté the spinach in the oiled pan—add a pinch of salt and pepper if desired.

5. After both have finished cooking; put them together in a bowl.

6. Transfer the olive oiled pan to the sausage fat pan—and add the eggs.

7. When the edges begin to cook—add the spinach, sausage, and cheese. Cook another minute—flip the omelet. Cook another two to three minutes.

8. Cover one pan with the other and let the combo steam.

9. Remove and enjoy your masterpiece!

10. *Serving Portion:* Fat: 43 g; Carbs 3 g; Protein: 31 g; Calories: 535

11. Lunch: Pancakes with Cream-Cheese Topping

12. Don't be alarmed, this is an excellent choice for any time and is so healthy.

13. *Ingredients*

14. 8 ¾ ounces cottage cheese

15. 5 eggs

16. 1 tablespoon ground psyllium husk powder

17. A pinch of salt

18. *For Frying:* Coconut oil or butter

19. *Ingredients for the Topping*

20. 2 tablespoons red or green pesto

21. ½ pound (8 ounces) ricotta or cream cheese

22. 2 tablespoons olive oil

23. Ground black pepper and Sea Salt

24. ½ thinly sliced red onion

25. *Instructions*

1. Combine one tablespoon of the olive oil with the pesto and cream cheese; set aside.

2. Using a hand blender, mix the salt, cottage cheese, eggs, and husk powder; blend until smooth. Let rest for ten minutes.

3. On the stovetop using the medium heat setting; heat two tablespoons of the oil or butter.

4. Drop several dollops of the cheese batter (2 to 3 inches in diameter), frying the pancakes a few minutes per side.

5. Serve with a few red onion slices with a drizzle of oil, pepper, and salt. You can also use fresh herbs, smoked fish roe or chopped chives.

6. **Dinner: Skillet Style Sausage and Cabbage Melt**

7. *Ingredients*

8. 4 spicy Italian chicken sausages

9. 2 tablespoons coconut oil

10. ½ cup diced onion

11. 1 ½ cups purple cabbage

12. 1 ½ cups green cabbage

13. 2 tablespoons chopped fresh cilantro

14. 2-1-ounce slices Colby jack cheese

15. *Instructions*

1. Start by removing the sausage casings and rough-chopping them. Shred the cabbage and chop the onions.

2. Add the coconut oil, cabbage, and onion in a large skillet using the med-high setting for approximately eight minutes (the veggies should be tender).

3. Blend the cheese and cover.

4. Turn the heat off and let it rest five minutes as the cheese melts.

5. When it is time to serve—stir gently and add the cilantro.

6. *Yields:* Four Servings

7. *Serving Portion*: 1: Fat: 14.62 g; Carbs 3.52 g; Protein: 18.26 g; Calories: 231

8. Day 7

9. Breakfast: Tapas

10. Have a great mixture!

11. *Ingredients*

12. Cold Cuts:

- Prosciutto

- Serrano ham

- Salami

- Chorizo

- Cheeses:

- Gouda

- Parmesan

- Mozzarella

- Cheddar

- Veggies:

- Pickled cucumbers

- Peppers

- Radishes

- Cucumbers

- Avocado with pepper and homemade mayonnaise

- Fresh Basil

- Splash of fresh squeezed lemon juice

- Nuts:

- Hazelnuts

- Almonds

- Walnuts

- *Instructions*

1. Cut all of the ingredients into cubes or sticks and split the avocado cutting its fruit into small wedges.

2. Blend with four ounces of mayonnaise pepper and maybe a splash of lemon juice

3. Use the avocado shells for the serving platter.

4. *Yields:* Four Servings

5. **Lunch: Tofu—Bok-Choy Salad**

6. *Tofu Ingredients:*

7. 15 ounces extra firm tofu

8. 2 teaspoons minced garlic

9. Juice from ½ a lemon

10. 1 tablespoon each:

- sesame oil

- water

- soy sauce

- rice wine vinegar

- *Bok Choy Salad Ingredients:*

- 2 tablespoons soy sauce

- 1 stalk green onion

- 2 tablespoons chopped cilantro

- 9 ounces bok choy

- 3 tablespoons coconut oil

- 1 tablespoon Sambal Olek

- Juice of ½ of a lime

- 1 tablespoon peanut butter

- 7 drops liquid Stevia

- *Instructions*

1. Press the tofu in towels for approximately five to six hours to dry.

2. Combine each of the marinade ingredients.

3. When dry; chop the tofu into squares and put in a plastic container/bag with the marinade sauce.

4. Leave it to sit for at least thirty minutes—preferably overnight.

5. Heat the oven to 350ºF. Bake for 30 to 35 minutes on a parchment paper-lined baking dish or a Silpat (non-stick baking sheet with a blend of fiberglass mesh and silicone).

6. In the interim, combine the dressing ingredients (except for the bok choy) in a mixing dish. Toss in the onion and cilantro.

7. Chop the bok choy as you would cabbage, into small slices.

8. Remove the tofu—combine, and enjoy.

9. *Note*: Bok choy is a Chinese vegetable.

10. *Serving Portion*: Fat: 35 g; Carbs 7.3 g; Protein: 25.0 g; Calories: 442.3

11. Dinner: Hamburger Stroganoff

12. *Ingredients*

13. 8 ounces sliced mushrooms

14. 1 pound ground beef

15. 2 minced cloves of garlic

16. 2 Tbsp. butter

17. 1 ¼ cups sour cream

18. 1/3 cup water or dry white wine

19. 1 tsp. lemon juice

20. ¼ tsp. paprika

21. 1 tsp. dried parsley

22. *Substitute*: You may also use one tablespoon fresh chopped parsley.

23. *Instructions*

1. Sauté the onions and garlic in a skillet prepared using one tablespoon of butter.

2. Mix in the beef into the pan— sprinkle with pepper and salt if desired. Cook until done and set to the side.

3. Use the remainder of the butter, the mushrooms, and the wine/water, and add them to the pan. Cook until half of the liquid is reduced and the mushrooms are soft.

4. Take them off the burner—add the paprika and sour cream.

5. On low heat stir in the meat and lemon juice.

6. Use additional spices for flavoring if desired.

7. *Serving Portion*: 1 (272 g): Fat: 28.1 g; Carbs 6.1 g; Protein: 38.7 g; Calories: 447

8. Day 8

9. Breakfast: Cheddar—Jalapeno Waffles

10. Ingredients

11. 3 large eggs

12. 1 small jalapeno

13. 3 ounces cream cheese

14. 1 tablespoon coconut flour

15. 1-ounce cheddar cheese

16. 1 teaspoon each:

- baking powder

- Psyllium husk powder

- *Instructions*

1. Combine all of the ingredients using an immersion blender (except for the jalapeno and cheese) until it has a smooth texture.

2. Add the cheese and jalapeno; blend and pour into the waffle iron.

3. You can garnish with your favorite ingredients in about five or six minutes total

4. *Note*: Psyllium husk is a native of Pakistan, Bangladesh, and India. It is available online at several locations

5. *Serving Portion:* 2 waffles: Fat: 28 g; Carbs 6 g; Protein: 16 g; Calories: 338

6. **Lunch: Salmon Tandoori with Cucumber Sauce**

7. *Ingredients*

8. 1 ½ Pounds Salmon (In pieces)

9. 2 tablespoons coconut oil

10. 1 tablespoon tandoori seasoning

11. *Ingredients for the Cucumber Sauce*

12. ½ cup shredded cucumber

13. 1 ¼ cup sour cream or mayonnaise

14. 2 minced garlic cloves

15. Juice of ½ of a lime

16. *Optional*: ½ teaspoon salt

17. *Ingredients for the Crispy Salad*

18. 3 ½ ounces arugula lettuce

19. 3 scallions

20. 1 yellow pepper

21. Juice of 1 lime

22. 2 avocados

23. *Instructions*

1. Preheat the oven to 350ºF.

2. Mix the tandoori seasoning and the 2 tablespoons of oil to coat the salmon.

3. Bake the salmon for fifteen to twenty minutes.

4. Combine the lime juice, garlic, cucumber (blot the water out with paper towels first), and sour cream/mayonnaise in a mixing dish.

5. Prepare the salad ingredients and enjoy.

6. *Yields*: Four Servings

7. **Dinner: Ground Beef Stir Fry**

8. *Ingredients*

9. 300 g (approximately 10 ½ ounces) ground beef

10. 5 medium brown mushrooms

11. ½ cup broccoli

12. 2 leaves kale

13. ½ medium Spanish onion

14. 1 Tbsp. coconut oil

15. ½ medium red pepper

16. 1 Tbsp. cayenne pepper

17. 1 Tbsp. Chinese Five Spices

18. *Note*: McCormick was used for the Five Spices

19. Instructions

1. Prepare the vegetables—slice the mushrooms —chop the broccoli.

2. Heat a frying pan on the stovetop using the med-high setting. Pour in the oil and toss in the onions. Cook for an additional minute.

3. Blend the remainder of the vegetables and cook an additional two minutes—stirring often.

4. Combine the spices and beef—lower the heat to medium—and continue cooking for approximately two more minutes.

5. Cover the pan and cook for five or ten more minutes until the beef is done.

6. *Serving Portion:* 1 (Recipe is for three servings): Fat: 18 g; Carbs 7 g; Protein: 29 g; Calories: 307

7. Day 9

8. Breakfast: Cheddar and Sage Waffles

9. Ingredients

10. 1 1/3 coconut flour

11. 1 teaspoon ground sage

12. ½ teaspoon salt

13. ¼ teaspoon garlic powder

14. 3 teaspoons baking powder

15. 2 cups canned coconut milk

16. ½ cup water

17. 3 tablespoons melted coconut oil

18. 1 cup shredded cheddar cheese

19. 2 eggs

20. *Instructions*

1. Prepare the waffle iron on the required manufacturer's setting. Grease the iron (top and bottom).

2. Blend all of the seasonings, flour, and baking powder in a container.

3. Mix the wet ingredients, stirring until the batter becomes stiff. Blend in the cheese.

4. Scoop out a one-third cup of the batter and place in each section of the iron.

5. Depending on how you like your waffles; you can run them through two cycles on the iron if you want it crispier.

6. *Serving Portion:* 1 waffles (The recipe serves 12): Fat: 17.21 g; Carbs 9.2 g; Protein: 6.52 g; Calories: 213.97

7. **Lunch: Crispy Shrimp Salad on an Egg Wrap**

8. *Ingredients for the Wraps*

9. 1-ounce butter

10. 4 eggs

11. Pepper and salt to taste

12. *Shrimp Salad Ingredients*

13. 6 ounces shrimp

14. 2 avocados

15. 1/2 of an apple/handful of radishes

16. 1 teaspoon lime juice

17. 1 celery stalk

18. 1 cup mayonnaise

19. 1 red chili pepper

20. 8 tablespoons fresh parsley or cilantro

21. *Instructions for the Wrap*

1. Cook and peel the shrimp. Finely chop the red chili pepper and fresh cilantro/parsley.

2. Whip the eggs with the pepper and salt.

3. Using a medium frying pan, melt the butter. Empty half of the egg batter until the egg gets firm, and repeat for the second one.

4. *Instructions for the Salad*

1. Slice the avocado and scoop out providing you with ½-inch cubes. Place them in a dish and give a fresh squeeze of juice over them and mix.

2. Dice the apple and thinly slice the celery, putting them with the avocado. Blend in the peppers, cilantro/parsley, and mayonnaise.

3. Combine well and gently stir in the shrimps. Add more salt if desired.

4. *Yields:* Two Servings

5. This is one of those meals that can be enjoyed with leafy greens or alone. Add a couple of boiled eggs in place of the wrap for another healthy choice.

6. **Dinner: Bacon Wrapped Meatloaf**

7. *Ingredients*

8. 1 finely chopped yellow onion

9. 1 ½ Pounds ground lamb, poultry, pork *or* beef

10. 2 tablespoons butter

11. 8 tablespoons heavy whipping cream

12. 1 egg

13. 6 ¾ tablespoons shredded cheese

14. 1 tablespoon dried basil/oregano

15. 1 tsp. salt

16. ½ tsp. black pepper

17. 7 ¾ ounces sliced bacon

18. *Optional:* ½ tablespoon tamari soy sauce

19. *For the Gravy:* 1 ¼ cups heavy whipping cream

20. *Instructions*

1. Preheat the oven to 400ºF/200ºC.

2. Saute the onion in a pan with the butter, but don't brown it.

3. Combine the meat in a container, adding all of the remainders of ingredients but omit the bacon. Don't over-work it, but blend the ingredients well, making a loaf.

4. Bake it in the center of the oven for approximately 45 minutes. You can use some aluminum foil to cover the meatloaf, just in case, the bacon begins to scorch.

5. Reserve any of the accumulated juices and make the gravy, blending it with the cream in a small saucepan.

6. Let the mixture come to a boil using low heat until it is creamy and the right texture, usually for approximately ten to fifteen minutes.

7. Spice it up with a drizzle of tamari soy sauce for a bit of flavor.

8. Have some cauliflower or broccoli on the side with some butter. It is all up to you to decide on the veggie choices.

9. *Yields*: Four Servings

10. Day 10

11. Breakfast: Omelet Wrap with Avocado & Salmon

12. *Ingredients*

13. 3 large eggs

14. ½ package smoked salmon (100 g or 1.8 ounces)

15. ½ avocado (3.5 ounces or 100 g)

16. 1 spring onion (1/2 ounce or 15 g)

17. 2 tablespoons cream cheese (full-fat—2.3 ounces or 64 g)

18. 2 tablespoons chives (freshly chopped)

19. 1 tablespoon butter or ghee

20. *Instructions*

1. In a mixing bowl—add a pinch of pepper and salt along with the eggs. Use a fork or whisk—mixing them well. Blend the chives and cream cheese.

2. Prepare the salmon and avocado (peel and slice).

3. In a sauté pan, melt the butter/ghee, and add the egg mixture. Cook until fluffy.

4. Put the omelet on a serving dish, and spoon the mixture of cheese over it.

5. Sprinkle the onion, prepared avocado, and salmon into the wrap.

6. Close and enjoy!

7. *Serving Portion*: Fat: 66.9g; Carbs 13.3 g; Protein: 36.9 g

8. Lunch: Tuna Avocado Melt

9. *Ingredients*

10. 1-10 - ounce can drained tuna

11. 1 medium cubed avocado

12. ¼ cup mayonnaise

13. 1/3 cup almond flour

14. ¼ teaspoon onion powder

15. ¼ cup parmesan cheese

16. ½ teaspoon garlic powder

17. 1/2 cup coconut oil (for frying)

18. *Instructions*

1. In a mixing container, blend all of the ingredients except for the coconut oil and avocado. Fold the cubed avocado into the tuna.

2. Make balls and coat each one with the almond flour.

3. Use the medium heat setting and put the oil in a pan—mix the tuna—and continue cooking until brown.

4. *Note*: Some people like to use this as a casserole dish.

5. *Yields*: Twelve Servings

6. *Per Serving Portion*: Fat: 11.8 g; Carbs 2.0 g; Protein: 6.2 g; Calories: 134.7

7. **Dinner: Hamburger Patties with Fried Cabbage**

8. *Ingredients for the Hamburger Patties*

9. 1 egg

10. 1 ½ Pounds ground beef

11. 3 ¼ ounces feta cheese

12. 1 tsp. salt

13. ¼ tsp. ground black pepper

14. 1 ¾ ounces finely- chopped, fresh parsley

15. 1-ounce butter

16. 1 tablespoon olive oil

17. *Ingredients for the Gravy*

18. 1 ¾ - Ounces fresh (coarsely chopped) parsley

19. 1 ¼ cups heavy whipping cream

20. Pepper and Salt

21. 2 tablespoons tomato paste

22. *Ingredients for the Green Cabbage*

23. 4 ¼ ounces butter

24. 1 ½ Pounds shredded green cabbage

25. Pepper and Salt

26. *Instructions*

1. Form eight oblong patties by blending all of the ingredients listed under the hamburger patties.

2. Using the med-high setting on the stovetop, prepare a skillet with olive oil and butter and fry the patties for a minimum of ten minutes.

3. Empty the whipping cream and tomato paste into the mixture—stir—and let them blend.

4. Serve with some parsley for garnishment.

5. *Instructions for Butter-fried Green Cabbage*

1. Use a food processor or knife to shred the cabbage.

2. Prepare a frying pan with the butter and sauté the cabbage for approximately fifteen minutes on the med-high setting.

3. Reduce the heat for the last five minutes (or so)—stirring regularly.

4. *Variations:* You can also enjoy this with whatever you desire, including spinach, carrots, mushrooms, acorn squash, or corn.

5. *Yields*: Four Servings

6. Day 11

7. Breakfast: The Breadless Breakfast Sandwich

8. *Ingredients*

9. 4 Eggs

10. 1-ounce ham/pastrami cold cuts

11. 2 tablespoons butter

12. 2 ounces of edam/provolone/cheddar cheese

13. Several drops of Worcestershire or Tabasco sauce

14. Pepper and salt to taste

15. *Instructions*

1. Cut the cheese into thick slices.

2. Prepare a frying pan over medium heat. Fry the eggs over-easy with a pinch of pepper and salt.

3. Add the choice of meat onto the two eggs, a layer of cheese, and the egg for the top of the 'bun.'

4. Give the sandwich a splash of Worcestershire sauce/Tabasco and serve. You can also use some French Dijon mustard to complement the ham.

5. *Yields:* Two Servings

6. **Lunch: Thai Fish With Coconut & Curry**

7. *Ingredients*

8. 1 ½ Pounds whitefish/salmon

9. 4 tablespoons butter/ghee

10. Pepper and salt

11. 1 to 2 tablespoons green/red curry paste

12. 8 tablespoons fresh chopped cilantro

13. 1 can coconut cream

14. 1 Pound broccoli/cauliflower

15. *For Greasing the Dish*: Olive oil/butter

16. *Instructions*

1. Grease a baking dish. Preheat the oven to 400ºF.

2. Place the salmon/fish in a dish where there is not any extra space between the dish and fish (not meant as a rhyme).

3. Place a dab of butter on each piece along with a shake of pepper and salt.

4. Combine the chopped cilantro, curry paste and coconut cream in a small container. Pour it over the fish.

5. Bake until the fish is falling apart done, usually about twenty minutes.

6. Boil the broccoli/cauliflower in water (lightly salted) for several minutes as a side dish.

7. *Yields*: Four Servings

8. **Dinner: Keto Tacos or Nachos**

9. *Ingredients*

10. 500 g or 17.6 ounces ground beef

11. 1 medium white onion (3.0 ounces)

12. 4 tacos

13. 1 teaspoon chili powder

14. 2 garlic cloves

15. ½ teaspoon ground cumin

16. 2 teaspoons extra-virgin coconut oil or ghee

17. 1 tablespoon unsweetened tomato puree

18. 1 cup water (8 ounces)

19. ½ teaspoon salt—more or less

20. Cayenne pepper or freshly ground black pepper

21. *Topping Ingredients*

22. 1 small head of lettuce (approximately 3.5 ounces or 100 g)

23. 1 cup or 5.3 ounces cherry tomatoes

24. 1 medium avocado (7.1 ounces or 200 g)

25. *Optional Toppings*

26. 4 tablespoons sour cream

27. 1 cup grated cheese

28. Veggies including cabbage, cucumbers, or peppers

29. *Instructions*

1. Using med-high, add some butter/ghee in a frying pan; toss in the onion. Sauté until brown and mix in the beef, continue cooking until the beef is done.

2. Add the cumin and chili powder. (You can substitute with 1 ½ teaspoon of paprika.)

3. Pour in the water and add the tomato puree. Also add pepper, and salt if you like for additional flavoring.

4. Continue cooking until the meat is done and approximately ¼ of the sauce is reduced. Set to the side and prepare the vegetable topping.

5. Use the meat mixture to stuff the shells. Garnish with some of the tomatoes, lettuce, and avocado.

6. As an option, you can add a bit of sour cream or cheddar cheese.

7. *Note*: You may use this as a tasty taco or on the side with the meat as the centerfold for the remainder of the veggies.

8. The choice is all yours!

9. **Day 12**

10. Breakfast: Scrambled Eggs With Halloumi Cheese

11. Ingredients

12. 5 to 6 eggs

13. 3 ½ ounces diced Halloumi cheese

14. 4 ½ ounces diced bacon

15. 8 tablespoons each:

- Pitted olives

- Chopped fresh parsley

- Pepper and Salt to taste

- 2 scallions

- 2 tablespoons olive oil

- *Instructions*

1. Dice the bacon and cheese.

2. Over the stovetop, use the medium-high setting; pour the oil into a frying pan. Add the scallions, cheese, and bacon—sauté until browned.

3. Whip/Whisk the eggs, pepper, salt, and parsley in a mixing container.

4. Pour the mixture into the pan over the cheese and bacon.

5. Reduce the heat—toss in the olives and sauté for several minutes.

6. All Ready! You can enjoy this with or without a salad.

7. *Yields*: Two Servings

8. Lunch: Salmon with Spinach and Chili Tones

9. *Ingredients*

10. 1 tablespoon chili paste

11. 1 ½ Pounds Salmon (in pieces)

12. 1 cup sour cream/mayonnaise

13. 1 ¾ cup olive oil/butter

14. 1 Pound fresh spinach

15. 4 tablespoons grated parmesan cheese

16. Pepper and Salt

17. Instructions

1. Place the oven setting to 400ºF/200ºC. Use some cooking oil to coat a baking dish/pan.

2. Flavor the salmon with the pepper and salt. Place in the dish skin side down.

3. Blend the chili paste, sour cream/mayonnaise, and parmesan cheese and spread it on the filets.

4. Bake until the salmon is done—usually fifteen to twenty minutes.

5. In the meantime, sauté the spinach until it wilts using the oil/butter.

6. *Yields*: Four Servings

7. **Dinner: Chicken Stuffed Avocado—Cajun Style**

8. *Ingredients*

9. 1 ½ cups cooked chicken (7.4 ounces or 210 g)

10. 2 medium or 1 large avocados (10.6 ounces or 300 g)

11. 2 tablespoons cream cheese/sour cream

12. 2 tablespoons lemon juice (fresh)

13. ¼ cup mayonnaise

14. ½ teaspoon each: onion powder & garlic powder

15. ¼ teaspoon each: salt and cayenne pepper

16. 1 teaspoon each: paprika and dried thyme

17. *Instructions*

1. Shred the chicken into small pieces.

2. Blend all of the ingredients—saving the salt and lemon juice until last.

3. Leave one-half to one-inch of the avocado flesh —scoop the middle. Remove the seeds.

4. Cut the center/scooped pieces of avocado into small pieces and fill each of the halves with the mixture of chicken.

5. *Yields*: Two Servings

6. *Serving Portion*: Fat: 50.6 g; Carbs 16.4 g; Protein: 34.5 g

7. Day 13
8.
9. Breakfast: Western Omelet

10. Ingredients

11. 2 tablespoons sour cream/heavy whipping cream

12. 6 eggs

13. Pepper and Salt

14. 2 ounces butter

15. 3 ½ ounces shredded cheese

16. 5 ounces of ham

17. ½ each:

- Finely chopped green bell peppers

- Finely chopped yellow onion

- *Instructions*

1. Whisk the sour cream/cream and eggs until fluffy. Flavor with the pepper and salt. Add half of the cheese and combine.

2. Melt the butter on the stovetop on the medium heat setting. Sauté the peppers, onions, and ham for just a few minutes.

3. Pour the batter in and fry until the omelet is almost firm.

4. Lower the heat and Sprinkle the remainder of the cheese on top of your masterpiece. Fold the omelet right away.

5. Have a fresh green salad as a perfect brunch touch!

6. *Yields*: Two Servings

7. **Lunch: Tortilla Ground Beef Salsa**

8. *Ingredients*

9. 1 ½ Pounds ground lamb/beef

10. 8 to 12 low-carb tortilla breads

11. 2 tablespoons olive oil

12. 1 cup of water

13. Tex-Mex seasoning (see below)

14. 1 teaspoon salt

15. Shredded leafy greens

16. 17 to 27 tablespoons shredded cheese

17. *Salsa Ingredients*

18. 1 to 2 diced tomatoes

19. 2 avocados

20. 1 tablespoon olive oil

21. Juice of 1 lime

22. 8 tablespoons fresh cilantro

23. Pepper and Salt

24. *Tex-Mex Seasoning*

25. 2 tsp. each:

- Paprika powder

- Chili powder

- 1 to 2 tsp. garlic/onion powder

- 1 tsp. ground cumin

- A pinch of cayenne pepper

- *Optional:* 1 tsp. salt

- *Instructions*

1. Prepare two batches of low-carb tortilla bread (see below).

2. Chop the cilantro. Take out the beef so it can become room temperature. Cold meats can have an effect on the cooking times, and it is more of a boil, not a fry.

3. On the stovetop, heat the oil using a large pan. Toss in the beef, and cook for around ten minutes.

4. Add the salt, water, and taco seasoning to the beef and simmer until most of the liquid has evaporated.

5. Meanwhile, prepare the salsa with all of the ingredients.

6. Serve on the tortilla bread with some shredded cheese along with the leafy greens.

7. *Yields*: Four Servings

8. **Low-Carb Tortillas**

9. *Ingredients*

10. 2 egg whites

11. 2 eggs

12. 6 ounces cream cheese

13. 1 tablespoon coconut flour

14. 1 to 2 teaspoons ground psyllium husk powder

15. ½ teaspoon salt

16. *Instructions*

1. Heat the oven to 400ºF. Prepare two baking sheets with parchment paper.

2. Whip the eggs and whites until fluffy. Blend in the cream cheese and whisk until creamy.

3. Combine the coconut flour, psyllium powder, and salt in a small container. Add the flour mixture for the batter a spoon at a time.

4. Spread out the batter on the baking tins, spreading thin, about ¼-inch thick. You can make two rectangles or four to six circles.

5. Bake until the tortilla begins to brown around the edges, usually about five minutes (or so).

6. Serve with some of your *Tex-Mex Ground Beef and Salsa.*

7. *Yields:* Two Servings

8. **Dinner: Fish Casserole with Mushrooms**

9. *Ingredients*

10. 1 Pound mushrooms

11. 3 ¼ ounces butter

12. 2 Tbsp. fresh parsley

13. 1 t. salt

14. Pepper (to taste)

15. 2 C. heavy whipping cream

16. 2 tablespoons fresh parsley

17. 2 to 3 Tbsp. Dijon mustard

18. 1 ½ Pounds white fish (Ex. Cod)

19. ½ Pound shredded cheese

20. 1 1/3 pounds cauliflower/broccoli

21. 3 ¼ ounces olive oil/butter

22. Instructions

1. Heat the oven to 350ºF. Lightly grease a baking dish for the fish.

2. Slice the mushrooms into wedges. Sauté in a pan with the butter, pepper, salt, and other herbs.

3. Empty the mustard and cream into the mixture and reduce the heat. Simmer for five to ten minutes until the sauce thickens.

4. Flavor the fish with the pepper and salt and add it to the prepared container. Sprinkle with ¾ of the cheese. Pour the creamed mushroom mixture over it and the rest of the cheese as a topping.

5. Bake approximately thirty minutes if the fish are frozen (less if not). After 20 minutes, test the fish to see if it flakes apart easily. Remember, the fish will cook for several minutes after it is removed from the oven.

6. Prepare the cauliflower into small florets, removing the leaves and stalks. You can use the entire broccoli by cutting it into rods/lengthwise.

7. Boil the veggie of choice, drain and add some butter/olive oil.

8. Coarsely mash with a fork or wooden spoon; adding some pepper and salt, and serve with your fish.

9. *Yields*: Four Servings

10. Day 14

11. Breakfast: Blueberry Smoothie

12. *Smoothie Ingredients*

13. 1 C. fresh or frozen blueberries

14. 1 2/3 C. coconut milk

15. 1 Tbsp. lemon juice

16. ½ tsp. vanilla extract

17. *Instructions*

1. Put all of the ingredients into a tall beaker. Mix using a hand mixer.

2. Pour the lemon juice in for additional flavoring.

3. *Notes:* You can substitute 1 ¼ cups of Greek yogurt for a dairy option and adjust with a small amount of water if you are searching for more liquid consistency. Add 1 tablespoon of a healthy oil such as coconut for more satiety.

4. *Yields:* Two Servings

5. **Lunch: Cheeseburger**

6. *Ingredients*

7. 7 ounces shredded cheese

8. 1 ½ Pounds ground beef

9. 2 teaspoons each:

- Onion powder

- Garlic powder

- Paprika

- *For Frying*

- 2 tablespoons fresh oregano

- Finely chopped butter

- *Salsa*

- 2 scallions

- 2 tomatoes

- 1 avocado

- Fresh Cilantro (to taste)

- Salt

- 1 tablespoon olive oil

- *Toppings*

- Lettuce

- Cooked bacon

- Dijon mustard

- Mayonnaise

- Pickled jalapenos

- Dill pickle

- *Instructions*

1. Chop all of the salsa ingredients in a small container and set to the side.

2. Combine all of the seasonings and ½ of the cheese into the beef mixture.

3. Prepare four burgers and grill or pan fry to your liking—adding cheese at the end of the cooking cycle.

4. Serve on the bed of lettuce with some mustard and a dill pickle.

5. *Yields*: Four Servings

6. Dinner: Turkey with Cream Cheese Sauce

7. *Ingredients*

8. 1 1/3 Pounds turkey breast

9. 2 tablespoons butter

10. 2 cups heavy whipping cream/sour cream

11. 7 ounces cream cheese

12. Pepper and salt

13. 1 tablespoon tamari soy sauce

14. 6 ¾ tablespoons small capers

15. *Instructions*

1. Heat the oven to 350ºF.

2. Sprinkle the turkey with pepper and salt for seasoning.

3. Add the butter to a frying pan. Sauté the turkey until golden. Place in the oven to finish cooking.

4. Using a small pan, combine the heavy cream/sour cream and cream cheese, bringing it to a boil; lower the heat and cook slowly for a few minutes.

5. On high heat in a small pan, use a small amount of butter or oil to fry the capers or enjoy them fresh.

6. When the turkey breast and veggies are done, add the sauce and capers on top of the turkey and serve along with some side dishes such as cauliflower or broccoli.

7. *Yields:* Four Servings

1. Combine all of the ingredients in a small mason jar or bowl.

2. Refrigerate overnight. It is ready when the seeds have gelled, and the pudding is thick.

3. Add some nuts and fresh fruit and 'dive in.'

4. **Cow-time Breakfast Skillet**

5. *Ingredients*

6. 2 medium diced sweet potatoes

7. 1 Pound breakfast sausage

8. 5 eggs

9. Handful of cilantro

10. 1 diced avocado

11. Hot sauce

12. *Optional:* Raw cheese

13. Pepper and Salt

14. *Instructions*

1. Heat the oven to 400ºF.

2. Use medium heat on the stovetop; place an iron or oven-safe skillet. Crumble and brown the sausage. Remove the sausage, cook the potatoes until crunchy, and reserve the grease.

3. Put the sausage back in the pan. Make some spaces in the 'wells' of the skillet, enough room for one egg. Crack the eggs into each of the wells.

4. Put the skillet into the preheated oven and bake enough for the eggs to set (about 5 minutes). Turn up the thermostat in the oven to the broil setting to let it broil the tops of the yolks with the crispy sweet potatoes.

5. Take the skillet out of the oven and cover it with some cilantro, avocado, and hot sauce.

6. Enjoy the tasty different flavors.

7. **Cream Cheese Pancakes**

8. *Ingredients for the Pancakes*

9. 2 oz. (room temperature) cream cheese

10. 2 organic eggs

11. ½ teaspoon cinnamon

12. 1 teaspoon granulated sugar substitute

13. *Instructions*

1. Place each of the pancake ingredients into a blender. Blend until creamy smooth; letting it rest for two minutes for the bubbles to settle back down.

2. Grease a pan with Pam spray or butter.

3. Pour about ¼ of the pancake batter into the hot pan; cooking for two minutes. Flip and continue cooking about one more minute.

4. Serve with berries or a sugar-free syrup of your choice.

5. *Yield*s: Four Pancakes

6. *Serving Size:* 1 Batch: Carbs 2.5 g net; Fat 29; Protein 17 g; Calories 344

7. Dairy-Free Latte

8. *Ingredients*

9. 2 Tbsp. coconut oil

10. 1 2/3 C. hot water

11. 2 eggs

12. 1 tsp. ground ginger/pumpkin pie spice

13. Splash of vanilla extract

14. *Instructions*

1. Use a stick blender to combine all of the ingredients.

2. If you want to replace the spices; you can use 1 tablespoon of instant coffee or cocoa.

3. Enjoy for a quick boost!

4. *Yields:* Two Servings

5. Keto Sausage Patties

6. *Ingredients*

7. 1 teaspoon maple extract

8. 2 tablespoons granular Swerve Sweetener

9. ½ teaspoon pepper

10. 1 pound ground pork

11. 2 tablespoons sage (chopped fresh)

12. 1/8 teaspoon cayenne

13. 1 teaspoon salt

14. ¼ teaspoon garlic powder

15. *Instructions*

1. Combine each of the ingredients in a large mixing container.

2. Shape the patties to about a one-inch thickness.

3. The recipe will make eight equal patties.

4. Add a small amount of olive oil or a dab of butter to a pan over medium heat. For each side, allow three to four minutes.

5. *Serving Portion:* 2 patties: Carbs 1.4 g; Fat: 11 g; Protein: 21 g; Calories: 187

6. **Keto Bacon**

7. *Use the Regular Oven*

1. Preheat to 350 ºF.

2. Put the bacon on a baking tray. Bake 20 to 25 minutes

3. Drain on a paper towel.

4. *Use the Microwave*

1. Put the bacon on paper towels in a single layer on a microwave-safe dish.

2. Use the high setting for four to six minutes.

3. *Use the Skillet*

1. Prepare the pan on the medium-low to medium.

2. Put the bacon into the pan single-layered.

3. Cook until the desired doneness is acquired.

4. *Serving Portion*: 2 slices: Fat: 19 g; Carbs 0.0

   g; Protein: 7 g; Calories: 200

5. Mushroom Omelet

6.

7. *Ingredients*

8. 3 eggs

9. 7/8 ounces shredded cheese

10. 2 to 3 mushrooms

11. Optional: 1/5 of an onion

12. Pepper and salt to taste

13. *For frying:* 7/8 ounces butter

14. *Instructions*

1. Whisk the eggs with the pepper and salt, add

the spices.

2. On the stovetop, use a frying pan to melt the

butter. Pour in the eggs.

3. When the omelet begins to cook to firmness; sprinkle the mushrooms, cheese, and onion on top.

4. Ease the edges up using a spatula, and fold in half. Remove from the pan when golden brown.

5. If you are having brunch; add a crispy salad.

6. *Yields:* One serving

7.

8.

9. Chapter 4: Additional Lunch and Dinner Recipes

10.

11. **Deviled Eggs**

12. With this tasty combination; it is hard to say breakfast or lunch; maybe brunch!

13. *Ingredients*

14. 6 large eggs

15. ¼ teaspoon yellow mustard

16. 1 tablespoon mayonnaise

17. 1 teaspoon paprika

18. *Garnish*: Parsley/salt/pepper

19. *Optional*

- ½ teaspoon cayenne pepper

- Several drops hot sauce

- 1 teaspoon cumin

- *Instructions*

1. Slice the eggs lengthwise.

2. Mix the egg yolks with the rest of the ingredients.

3. Put the goodies inside the egg bed.

4. Sprinkle with condiments as desired.

5. *Serving Portion:* Fat: 20 g; Carbs 1 g; Protein: 19 g; Calories: 265

6. **Ham and Apple Flatbread**

7. *Crust Ingredients*

8. ¾ cup almond flour

9. 2 cups grated mozzarella cheese (part-skim)

10. 2 tablespoons cream cheese

11. 1/8 teaspoon dried thyme

12. ½ teaspoon sea salt

13. *Topping Ingredients*

14. 4 ounces sliced ham (low-carb)

15. ½ small red onion

16. 1 cup grated Mexican cheese

17. ¼ medium apple

18.   1/8 teaspoon dried thyme

19.   *Instructions*

1. Remove the seeds and core from the apples. You can leave them unpeeled but will need to use a vegetable peeler to make the thin slices.

2. Heat the oven to 425ºF.

3. Cut two pieces of parchment paper to fit into a 12-inch pizza pan (approximately two inches larger than the pan).

4. Use the high-heat setting and place a double boiler (water in the bottom pan), and bring the water to boiling. Lower the heat setting and add the cream cheese, mozzarella cheese, salt, thyme, and almond flour to the top of the double boiler—stirring constantly.

5. When the cheese mixture resembles dough, place it on one of the pieces of parchment—and knead the dough until totally mixed.

6. Roll the dough into a ball—placing it at the center of the paper—place the second piece of paper over the top, and roll with a rolling pin (or a large glass).

7. Place the dough onto the pizza pan (leaving the paper connected).

8. Poke several holes in the dough and put into the preheated oven for approximately six to eight minutes.

9. When browned, remove it, and lower the setting of the oven to 350ºF.

10. Arrange the cheese, apple slices, onion slices, and ham pieces.

11. Top off with the remainder (3/4 cup) of cheese.

12. Season with the ground pepper, salt, and thyme.

13. Place the finished product into the oven, baking until you see a golden brown crust.

14. Slide it from the parchment paper and cool two or three minutes before cutting.

15. *Yields*: Eight Slices

16. *Tip*: If you do not own a double boiler; you can substitute with a mixing dish over a pot of boiling water as a substitute.

17. *Serving Portion*: 1: Fat: 20 g; Carbs 5 g; Protein: 16 g; Calories: 255

18. Chicken Breast with Herb Butter

19. *Ingredients for the Fried Chicken*

20. 4 Chicken Breasts

21. Pepper and Salt

22. 1-ounce of olive oil/butter

23. *Herb Butter Ingredients*

24. 1 clove garlic

25. 1/3 Pound butter (room temperature)

26. 1 tsp. lemon juice

27. ½ tsp. each:

- garlic powder

- salt

- 4 Tbsp. fresh chopped parsley

- *Leafy Greens*

- ½ Pound leafy greens (baby spinach for example)

- *Instructions*

1. Take the butter out of the refrigerator for at least thirty to sixty minutes before you begin to prepare your meal.

2. Add all of the ingredients, including the butter, and blend thoroughly in a small container; set to the side.

3. Use the pepper and salt to flavor the chicken. Cook the chicken filets in a skillet using the butter over medium heat. To avoid dried out filets, lower the temperature the last few minutes.

4. Serve over a bed of greens with some melted herb butter over the top.

5. *Yields*: Four Servings

6. **Low-Carbonara**

7. *Ingredients*

8. 2/3 Pounds diced Pancetta/bacon

9. 1 ¼ cups heavy whipping cream

10. 1 tablespoon butter

11. 3 1/3 tablespoons mayonnaise

12. Fresh chopped parsley

13. Pepper and salt

14. 2 Pounds zucchini

15. 3 ½ ounces grated Parmesan cheese

16. 4 egg yolks

17. *Instructions*

1. Empty the heavy cream into a saucepan, bringing it to a boil. Lower the burner and continue boiling until the juices are reduced by about a third.

2. Fry the bacon/pancetta; reserve the fat.

3. Combine the heavy cream, mayonnaise, pepper, and salt into the saucepan mixture.

4. Make 'zoodles' out of the zucchini using a potato peeler or spiralizer.

5. Add the zoodles to the warm sauce and serve with egg yolks, bacon, parsley, and freshly grated cheese.

6. Drizzle a bit of the bacon grease on top.

7. Yummy!

8. *Yields:* Four Servings

9. **Pesto Chicken Casserole with Olives and Cheese**

10. *Ingredients*

11. 1 ½ Pounds chicken breasts/thighs

12. 3 ½ ounces green or red pesto

13. 8 tablespoons pitted olives

14. 1 2/3 cups heavy whipping cream

15. ½ Pound diced feta cheese

16. Pepper and Salt

17. 1 finely chopped garlic clove

18. *For Frying*: Butter

19. *For Serving*

- Olive oil

- 1/3 Pound leafy greens

- Sea salt

- *Instructions*

1. Heat the oven to 400ºF.

2. Cut the chicken into pieces and flavor with the pepper and salt.

3. Place in a skillet with the butter, cooking until well done.

4. Combine the heavy cream and pesto.

5. Put the chicken pieces in the baking dish with the garlic, feta cheese, and olives, along with the pesto mix.

6. Bake for 20 to 30 minutes until the perfect color.

7. Enjoy with some green beans, sautéed asparagus, or another veggie of your choice.

8. *Yields*: Four Servings

9. Red Pesto Pork Chops

10. *Ingredients*

11. 4 Pork chops

12. 4 tablespoons red pesto

13. 2 tablespoons olive oil/butter

14. 6 tablespoons mayonnaise

15. *Instructions*

1. Thoroughly rub the chops with the pesto.

2. Fry on medium heat in a skillet with oil/butter for eight minutes. Reduce the heat and simmer four more minutes.

3. Serve with the pesto mayonnaise: 6 tablespoons of mayonnaise (+) 1 to 2 tablespoons pesto.

4. Serve with a large salad. You can also add a serving of cauliflower and broccoli with cheese.

5. Chapter 5:
6. Snacks and Desserts for the Diet Plan
7.

8. **Keto Ginger Snap Cookies**

9. Ingredients

10. ¼ cup unsalted butter

11. 1 large egg

12. 2 C. almond flour

13. ½ tsp. ground cinnamon

14. 1 tsp. vanilla extract

15. 1 C. sugar substitute/Erythritol (Swerve)

16. 2 tsp. ground ginger

17. ¼ tsp. each:

- Salt

- Ground cloves

- Nutmeg

- *Instructions*

1. Set the oven to 350ºF.

2. Combine the dry ingredients in a small dish.

3. Combine the remainder components to the dry mixture, and mix using a hand blender/mixer. (The dough will be crumbly and stiff.)

4. Measure out the dough for each cookie and flatten with a fork or your fingers.

5. Bake for approximately nine to eleven minutes or till they are browned.

6. *Yields:* 24 Cookies

7. **Pumpkin Pudding**

8. *Ingredients*

9. ¼ cup pumpkin puree

10. 1/3 cup granulated (Erythritol/Stevia)

11. ½ tsp. pumpkin pie spices

12. 1 tsp. xanthan gum

13. 3 medium egg yolks

14. 1 ½ cups whipping cream

15. 1 tsp. vanilla extract

16. *For the Cream Mixture*

17. 3 Tbsp. granulated stevia

18. 1 cup whipping cream

19. ½ tsp. vanilla extract

20. *Instructions*

1. Blend the pumpkin spice, xanthan gum, sweetener, and salt. Whip/whisk until the texture is smooth. Add the yolks, puree, and vanilla extract to the mixture; blend thoroughly.

2. Slowly pour in the whipping cream, after all of the cream is added. Using medium heat let the mixture come to a boil.

3. Continue the process for about 4 to 7 minutes, until thickened.

4. Place in the refrigerator in a container. Stir every ten minutes.

5. Meanwhile, in a medium dish, use a mixer to whip the one cup of whipping cream resulting in stiff peaks. Add the vanilla and sweetener; stir gently.

6. After the base pudding mixture has cooled; fold the whipped cream into the mix.

7. Scoop the pudding into small serving dishes and chill for a minimum of one to two hours.

8. *Note*: The Xanthan gum is available on Amazon.

9. *Yields*: Six Servings

10. No-Bake Cashew Coconut Bars

11. *Ingredients*

12. ¼ cup maple syrup/sugar-free

13. 1 cup almond flour

14. ¼ cup melted butter

15. 1 teaspoon cinnamon

16. ½ cup cashews

17. A pinch of salt

18. 1/4 cup shredded coconut

19. *Instructions*

1. Combine the flour and melted butter in a large mixing dish.

2. Add the maple syrup, cinnamon, salt, and coconut—blend well.

3. Use roasted or raw cashews. Chop them and add to the cashew-coconut bar dough. Blend well again.

4. Cover a cookie pan with parchment paper and spread the dough onto the paper in an even layer.

5. Place in the fridge for a minimum of two hours. Slice them and enjoy!

6. *Yields:* Eight Servings

7. **Brownie Cheesecake**

8. *The Brownie Base Ingredients*:

9. 2 ounces chopped unsweetened chocolate

10. 2 large eggs

11. ½ cup butter

12. 1/2 cup almond flour

13. 1 pinch of salt

14. ¼ cup cocoa powder

15. ¾ cup granulated Erythritol/Swerve Sweetener

16. ¼ cup pecans/walnuts (chopped)

17. ¼ teaspoon vanilla

18. *Cheesecake Filling Ingredients*

19. 2 large eggs

20. 1 pound softened cream cheese

21. ½ cup granulated sugar/Swerve sweetener

22. ½ teaspoon vanilla extract

23. ¼ cup heavy cream

24. *Instructions*

1. Butter a nine-inch springform pan; wrapping the bottom with foil.

2. Set the oven at 325ºF.

3. Melt the chocolate and butter in a microwave-safe dish for 30 seconds.

4. Whisk the cocoa powder, almond flour, and salt in a small dish.

5. In a separate dish; whip the vanilla, eggs, and Swerve until smooth.

6. Blend the flour mixture and chocolate/butter mixture. Blend in the nuts.

7. Spread out in the prepared dish and bake for approximately 15 to 20 minutes.

8. Let it cool for about 20 to 25 minutes.

9. *For the Filling*

1. Reduce the oven setting to 300ºF.

2. Blend the Swerve, the vanilla, cream, eggs, and cream cheese in a mixing container until everything is thoroughly mixed. Empty the

filling ingredients into the crust and place it on a large cookie sheet.

3. Bake for about 35 to 45 minutes. The center should barely jiggle.

4. Loosen the edges with a knife.

5. Place them in the fridge for a minimum of three hours.

6. *Yields:* Ten Servings

7. **Chocolate Soufflé**

8. *Ingredients*

9. 1/3 cup sugar substitute (Lakanto Mont Fruit/ Amazon)

10. 1 tablespoon butter

11. 6 large egg whites

12. 3 large egg yolks

13. 5 ounces unsweetened chocolate

14. *Note*: The eggs work best at room temperature.

15. *Instructions*

1. Preset the oven to 375ºF.

2. Use the butter to grease a soufflé dish.

3. Use a double boiler or a metal dish above a pan of boiling water to melt the chocolate. (Stir the mix constantly.)

4. Remove the dish and whip in the yolks until the mix hardens. Set it to the side.

5. Use a pinch of salt, whip/whisk the egg whites with an electric mixer on the highest setting.

6. Gradually, blend in the sugar/Lakanto. Continue until you see stiff peaks.

7. Stir in one cup of the egg whites into the chocolate combination folding gently using a silicone spatula. Pour the mixture into the soufflé dish.

8. Bake approximately twenty minutes. The center should still jiggle with the soufflé crusted and puffed on the top.

9. Serve this delicious treat right away.

10. *Topping/Optional*: Coconut whipped cream

11. *Yields*: Four Treats

12. *Note*: To make the soufflé rise evenly; use your thumb to remove the batter from the top of the dish.

13. Macaroon Keto Bombs

14. Your curiosity is wondering, "What is a bomb?" The reasoning is that this is good for you and is too delicious to pass by when you are craving a treat!

15. *Ingredients*

16. ½ cup shredded coconut

17. ¼ cup almond flour

18. 2 tablespoons sugar substitute (Swerve)

19. 3 egg whites

20. 1 tablespoon each:

- Coconut oil

- Vanilla extract

- *Instructions*

1. Set the oven at 400ºF.

2. In a small container, combine the almond flour, coconut, and Swerve.

3. Use a small saucepan to melt the coconut oil. Add the vanilla extract.

4. *Note*: To mount the egg whites, place a medium dish in the freezer.

5. Add the oil to the flour mixture and blend well.

6. Break the egg whites in the cold dish and whip until stiff peaks are formed. Blend the egg whites into the flour mixture.

7. Spoon the mixture into a muffin cup or place them on a baking sheet.

8. Bake the macaroons for eight minutes or until you see browned edges.

9. Cool the bombs before you attempt to remove them from the pan.

10. *Yields*: Ten Servings

11. Conclusion

12.

13. Thank for viewing your personal copy of the *Ketogenic Diet: Better Energy, Performance, and Natural Fuel to Good Health for the Smart.* Let's hope it was informative and able to provide you with all of the tools you need to achieve your goals as a better energy management specialist.

14. The next step is to test some of the recipes for yourself and discover what you have been missing since you have tried so many times unsuccessfully using other dieting methods. The recipes provided have been tested by qualified chefs who know the deal when it comes to energy performance.

15. Just remember, making advances towards a better lifestyle begins at the breakfast, lunch, and dinner table. You can supplement as you see fit once you have the knack of how the

balance works.

- Lunch: Chicken—Broccoli—Zucchini Boats
- Dinner: Steak-Lovers Slow-Cooked Chili
- **Day 5**
- Breakfast: Brownie Muffins
- Lunch: Bacon-Avocado-Goat Cheese Salad
- Dinner: Tenderloin Stuffed Keto Style
- **Day 6**
- Breakfast: Sausage—Feta—Spinach Omelet
- Lunch: Pancakes with Cream-Cheese Topping
- Dinner: Skillet Style Sausage and Cabbage Melt
- **Day 7**
- Breakfast: Tapas
- Lunch: Tofu—Bok-Choy Salad
- Dinner: Hamburger Stroganoff
- **Day 8**
- Breakfast: Cheddar—Jalapeno Waffles
- Lunch: Salmon Tandoori with Cucumber Sauce
- Dinner: Ground Beef Stir Fry

- **Day 9**

  - Breakfast: Cheddar and Sage Waffles

  - Lunch: Crispy Shrimp Salad on an Egg Wrap

  - Dinner: Bacon Wrapped Meatloaf

- **Day 10**

  - Breakfast: Omelet Wrap with Avocado & Salmon

  - Lunch: Tuna Avocado Melt

  - Dinner: Hamburger Patties with Fried Cabbage

- **Day 11**

  - Breakfast: The Breadless Breakfast Sandwich

  - Lunch: Thai Fish With Coconut & Curry

  - Dinner: Keto Tacos or Nachos

- **Day 12**

  - Breakfast: Scrambled Eggs With Halloumi Cheese

  - Lunch: Salmon with Spinach and Chili Tones

  - Dinner: Chicken Stuffed Avocado—Cajun Style

CPSIA information can be obtained
at www.ICGtesting.com
Printed in the USA
LVHW041237301020
670162LV00003B/73

9 789814 950336